THORSONS
PRINCIPLES
OF

HYPNOTHERAPY

VERA PEIFFER

Thorsons
An Imprint of HarperCollins*Publishers*

Thorsons
An Imprint of HarperCollins*Publishers*
77–85 Fulham Palace Road,
Hammersmith, London W6 8JB
1160 Battery Street
San Francisco, California 94111–1213
Published by Thorsons 1996

5 7 9 10 8 6 4

© Vera Peiffer 1996

Vera Peiffer asserts the moral right to
be identified as the author of this work

A catalogue record for this book
is available from the British Library

ISBN 0 7225 3242 3

Printed and bound in Great Britain by
Clays Ltd, St Ives plc

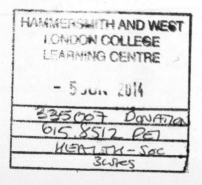

FOR URSULA MARKHAM
WITH LOVE AND THANKS
FOR GETTING ME STARTED

The definition of hypnosis used in
Chapter 2 of this book has been quoted with
permission from the *Encyclopaedia Britannica*,
15th edition (1990), vol. 6, p. 203.

CONTENTS

ACKNOWLEDGEMENTS

T he publishers would like to thank Jillie Collings for her suggestion for the title of this series, *Principles of...*

INTRODUCTION

With demand for complementary therapies growing by up to 30 per cent a year, the UK's Health Education Authority (HEA) recently commissioned a book which offers a general guide to complementary medicine and therapies. In this book complementary therapies are rated according to their popularity, their medical credibility, their scientific validity and their availability. Together with acupuncture and osteopathy, hypnotherapy achieved the highest rating in all four categories.

Despite its popularity and proven effectiveness, hypnotherapy has at times come into the spotlight in a negative way. Stage shows, sensationalist reports and the unethical conduct of a small number of therapists have added to the confusion that still exists about this ancient form of therapy. Even though most people nowadays have heard about hypnotherapy, general knowledge about the subject does not usually go beyond the use of suggestions to help people stop smoking or lose weight. Yet there is a lot more that hypnotherapy can do.

Principles of Hypnotherapy sums up scientific findings about hypnosis and explains how hypnosis is used to help with various conditions such as depression, anxiety, panic attacks, pain control, lack of confidence and many more. You will find clear descriptions not only of the workings of hypnotherapy, illustrated by case histories, but also a list of things you should look out for if you are thinking of visiting a hypnotherapist.

A whole section is devoted to False Memory Syndrome, and you will find advice on what questions to ask to avoid ending up with a practitioner who might lead you into false memories.

HISTORY & DEVELOPMENT OF HYPNOSIS

As a great number of ancient documents verify, hypnosis is one of the oldest therapies. Cuneiform writings that date back to four thousand years before Christ reveal that the Sumerians used hypnosis as a therapeutic tool. Specially trained priest-doctors gave sufferers hypnotic suggestions, as did the later Hindu fakirs, the Persian magi and the Indian yogi. The Ebers papyrus tells us that in ancient Egypt, priest-doctors would ask sufferers to fix their gaze on a glossy piece of metal to induce a hypnotic trance – a precursor of the 'fixation technique' (*see page 92*) which is still in use today in modern hypnotherapy.

The use of hypnotic suggestions for healing was employed all the way into the Middle Ages, but it was not until 1530 that an explanation other than divine intervention was offered for the cures achieved by hypnosis.

Paracelsus (1493 – 1541), a scientist and physician of Swiss origin, developed a theory about the interrelationship between the stars and human disease processes, and also about the magnetic powers man has over man. Later, Franz Anton Mesmer (1734 – 1815), an Austrian physician, developed the theory further by assuming that there was a universal fluid which enveloped and pervaded the earth and all human beings, and that the planets could bring about change in the human body through this invisible magnetic fluid. Mesmer named the fluid 'animal magnetism' and suggested that disease or pain arose from an unbalanced distribution of this fluid in the sufferer's body. He posited that magnets, with their power to attract and repel, could help rebalance this fluid. Healing by touch and healing by stroking were other methods used at the time, and Mesmer decided to combine all these measures in order to cure his patients. Mesmer would have his patients hold a piece of metal to the diseased or painful part of their bodies; and while they did so he would touch their bodies with a metal rod, claiming that this would redistribute the magnetic fluid and thereby facilitate a cure.

Mesmer was a charismatic man who set the scene for his patients by leading them into a darkened room where he would have music playing to create the appropriate atmosphere. In the middle of the room stood an oak tub filled with iron filings, powdered glass and water, from which emerged iron rods. Patients had to observe strict silence as they walked in and sat around the tub so that they could hold the metal rods while Mesmer made a dramatic entrance, cloak flowing, walking among the patients and occasionally touching one of them with his hand or his metal rod. During this process the patients would often show physical reactions such as coughing or convulsions. These reactions were called 'crises' and were regarded as signs that healing was taking place.

Mesmer achieved spectacular results in many cases where conventional doctors had been unable to help. This angered his medical colleagues and he was forced to flee from Vienna to Paris, but his problems followed him there. Instigated by the medical profession, King Louis XVI ordered an investigation into 'animal magnetism'. When no scientific proof could be found to explain the cures, this type of therapy was prohibited.

Even the mere discussion of the subject could led to withdrawal of permission to practise as a doctor. Mesmer's cures were consequently explained as being merely the result of his patients' imagination. Mesmer had to stop practising and went back to his birthplace, where he died in 1815.

In 1813, Abbé Faria (1755 – 1819) corrected Mesmer's theory by stating that, according to research he had conducted in India, there was no need for a universal fluid to induce trance – it was the power of suggestion that achieved the sleeplike state. This new theory was also supported by Alexandre Bertrand, an eminent French physician, who added that it was not so much the person who gave the suggestions but the influence of the patient's imagination that brought about results.

The induction of 'lucid sleep' was developed further by the English optometrist James Braid (1795 – 1860). After seeing the Swiss 'magnetizer' Lafontaine, Braid attempted to expose him as a charlatan. However, on experimenting with various people, including his own relatives and servants, Braid found that the trancelike state was quite genuine and that people could go into this state quite naturally after fixing their gaze on a shiny object for just a few minutes. He named this state hypnosis, after the Greek word *hypnos*, meaning sleep. Braid found that fixation resulted in hypnosis for both people and animals alike. He obtained excellent results in medical and surgical cases and consequently offered to read a paper on the subject to the British Association for the Advancement of Science, but his offer was rejected. A similar reaction was encountered by other physicians who had used hypnosis successfully in their work – they were either ignored, ridiculed or dismissed from their professional posts.

It was only when Professor Hippolyte Bernheim (1843 – 1919) became interested in the work of Ambroise-Auguste Liébeault, a Parisian physician who had been using hypnotic suggestions successfully for many years, that hypnosis started to be taken more seriously by the medical establishment. Professor Bernheim, a famous neurologist from Nancy, was so impressed by what he saw at Liébeault's clinic that he founded the School of Nancy, thereby creating the first institute for the scientific application of hypnosis. In 1886, Bernheim published his book *De La Suggestion* (About Suggestion) which laid the foundation upon which modern suggestion therapy is based.

At around the same time, Doctor Joseph Breuer, a Viennese physician, discovered by chance that if he encouraged his patients to speak freely in hypnosis they could recall events which they could not remember in a normal state. As a consequence of recalling repressed traumatic events, the patients experienced an emotional reaction (not unlike Mesmer's 'crisis') which resulted in the alleviation of their symptoms. Sigmund Freud (1856 – 1939) worked with Breuer and based some of his work on Breuer's findings, although he later abandoned hypnosis because he found that he was sometimes unable to overcome his patients' resistance to releasing traumatic memories. But even though Freud ultimately left hypnosis behind to concentrate on the development of his psychoanalytical approach, hypnosis continued to enjoy steady progress. During and after the First World War, hypnosis was applied increasingly to help soldiers overcome the trauma they had experienced in the trenches.

In 1953, a subcommittee to the British Medical Association's Psychological Group Committee was founded which started investigating hypnosis as an adjunct to medicine. A great deal has been discovered since then about the workings and functions of the subconscious mind and how it influences the way human beings react and behave. The subcommittee found that hypnosis was a very useful tool when it came to treating psychosomatic and psychoneurotic illnesses, as well as being of great help in surgery, dentistry and obstetrics as a pain-reliever. The committee also suggested that the subject of hypnosis should be included in the training of psychiatrists.

Today, hypnosis is used successfully not only in surgery and dentistry and as a psychotherapeutic tool, but in many areas of personal development such as increasing performance in a particular sport or career, and raising a person's level of confidence and competence in everyday life by enhancing memory, improving study habits, releasing blocked potential and instilling a more positive attitude.

WHAT IS HYPNOSIS?

The new *Encyclopaedia Britannica* (15th edition) defines hypnosis as:

> a special psychological state with certain physiological attributes, resembling sleep only superficially and marked by a functioning of the individual at a level of awareness other than the ordinary conscious state. This state is characterized by a degree of increased receptiveness and responsiveness in which inner experiential perceptions are given as much significance as is generally given only to external reality.

This is an accurate general description of the state of hypnosis. But what happens on a physical level when someone is in hypnosis? How does the person in hypnosis experience this state? And what is happening in the mind during hypnosis?

Before we look at scientific research and individual experience of hypnosis, it is necessary to understand some basics about the human mind.

THE CONSCIOUS AND SUBCONSCIOUS MIND

The mind, just like an iceberg, consists of two parts: the tip of the iceberg – that is, the conscious mind which helps us with daily decision-making processes and also assists us in new situations where we have to apply rational thinking to fathom out what to do and how to do it – and the hidden depths of the iceberg – the subconscious mind, which works on 'auto-pilot' and deals with a variety of tasks, such as:

- the emotions

- imagination

- memories

- the autonomic nervous system.

THE EMOTIONS

Emotions are the opposite of rationality. Emotions such as joy, happiness, anger, disappointment, fear and so on come up without us 'planning' to have them; they are 'just there'. A thought in our minds can provoke an emotion, as can a remark someone makes in our presence or even a remark someone made many years ago.

IMAGINATION

The term 'imagination' is used here as an umbrella term for a number of other facets of the subconscious mind, such as ideas, creativity, intuition, premonition, fantasies, daydreaming and dreaming.

MEMORIES

The subconscious mind holds memories of everything we have ever seen, heard, experienced or learned. This does not necessarily mean that we have total access to that information; a lot of it will normally stay buried in our subconscious, although hypnosis can considerably facilitate recall.

The autonomic nervous system controls and regulates our internal organs automatically. For example, it makes the skin contract ('goosebumps') when we step out into the cold; it automatically dilates the pupils when the light gets dim and contracts them again when the light gets brighter. The autonomic nervous system will also make your mouth water when you are looking at or even just thinking about a delicious dish.

Those four main functions of the subconscious work closely together, and an automatic cycle is established. If, for example, someone tells you off or criticizes you repeatedly in a harsh or unfair way, your subconscious releases unpleasant emotions and they in turn trigger a stressed physical reaction via the autonomic nervous system – your heart starts beating a little faster because adrenalin gets pumped into the bloodstream, your blood-pressure goes up and your blood sugar level rises. This unpleasant emotional and physical feeling will then influence your memory, leaving a negative 'memory trace' in connection with the person who just criticized you. When you think about that person afterwards, you may find yourself reliving the event again and again, in this way deepening the negative memory trace. As a consequence, when you are due to see that person again you may well find that you experience the same negative emotional and physical reactions, even before the meeting takes place.

An example of positive input would be if, for example, a little girl comes in contact with a dog for the first time. If she is gently encouraged to stroke the animal and the dog responds in a friendly manner, the child will have a pleasant feeling inside, her body relaxes and she takes away with her a happy memory of that dog. A positive memory trace has now been established, and with the help of further similarly positive experiences the child's future reaction to dogs is likely to be relaxed and free of fear.

We all carry positive and negative memory traces with us which come from past experiences, and we react to any given situation according to these memories.

Many memory traces go all the way back into childhood, although we do not necessarily consciously recall the original incident. However, we often still experience the same feeling that went with the original event as soon as we encounter a similar situation later in life. We may have forgotten that we were bitten by a dog as a child, but our subconscious will 'remind' us of the incident indirectly by emitting a feeling of fear whenever we see a dog.

Feelings do not overcome us out of the blue; they are always linked to a real incident. The stronger the feeling that accompanies an event, the more likely it is that it will produce a strong memory trace and result in an automatic, spontaneous reaction to future similar events. Hypnosis can help to uncover the original, triggering event and thereby helps to break the pattern of negative responses we may have to certain events, people or situations.

SCIENTIFIC FINDINGS

Over the last few decades hypnosis has become increasingly recognized as a valuable therapeutic tool, not just by the public but also by the medical profession. As a consequence, research funds have been made available to run clinical tests to investigate the workings of hypnosis. Most research still comes from the US, but tests under laboratory conditions have also been carried out in Canada, Australia, Germany and other European countries.

Research has focused on a variety of physical functions which are measured before, during and after hypnosis. It has been found that, while a subject is in hypnosis, the breathing rate and heart beat slow down, the bronchi of the lungs dilate, blood-pressure drops and the production of stomach acid is reduced. In addition, no stress hormones are released into the bloodstream. Scientists at the University of Constance have observed that, even in subjects in only a light trance, white blood cells cling more firmly to blood vessels, which is thought to increase the body's immune efficiency. The body also seems to produce more of these immune-enhancing lymphocytes while under hypnosis, which could explain why hypnosis has been used successfully in the treatment of cancerous cells.

These scientific findings make it clear why hypnosis (used either as self-hypnosis or induced by a therapist) is an ideal tool to help alleviate physical problems such as asthma, tension headaches, stomach disorders, high blood-pressure and many other stress-related problems.

Thanks to further research carried out over recent years, it has now also been shown that hypnosis is not the same thing as sleep. Scientists at Stanford University in California tested the brain waves of hypnotized subjects, using an electroencephalograph (EEG), an apparatus which records the electrical activity of the brain. As the nerve cells of the brain generate rhythmic electrical impulses, the EEG records these as peaks and troughs on a line graph. In hypnosis the brain emits *alpha waves*, which denote a mentally alert but physically relaxed state. This contrasts strongly with the type of waves emitted when the subject is actually asleep; in this case, the waves become extremely slow, proving that sleep is a very different state to a hypnotic trance – a reassuring finding for anyone who is concerned about becoming 'unconscious' during hypnosis.

WHAT IT FEELS LIKE TO BE IN HYPNOSIS

There are still various myths and misconceptions that circulate in the public mind about hypnosis. Many people are still scared of experiencing hypnosis because they assume that they will be unconscious or a helpless zombie, at the beck and call of the dubious intentions of the hypnotherapist. This is not so. In reality, being in hypnosis is quite unspectacular.

Hypnosis is a natural phenomenon which we encounter daily. Have you ever found yourself:

- looking out of the window with a far-away look in your eyes, thinking intently about a particular thing?

- reading a really good book and getting so absorbed in it that you forget where you are while you are reading?

- getting involved in a lengthy but pleasurable task like gardening or playing a computer game and forgetting about the time?

- driving along, or sitting on a train for a long time and feeling that the monotony of the journey is nearly putting you to sleep?

- jogging or working out and feeling detached from your worries for a while?

- at a rock or pop concert and feeling high afterwards without having smoked or drunk alcohol?

If you can relate to any of these experiences, you have already been in hypnosis; the only difference is that you would not call it hypnosis in everyday terms. You would probably call the sensation 'daydreaming', 'being far away with your thoughts' or 'high'. When you are staring out of your window as you are daydreaming, you still know that you are sitting in your living room, but this information is not very important while you are in the process of pursuing your thoughts. However, if anything needs your attention, if someone calls your name or the phone starts ringing, you snap out of your daydream immediately. And if someone happened to be watching you while you were daydreaming and were later to suggest that you had been out of control or unconscious, you would no doubt dismiss this as nonsense, and quite rightly so.

We all switch in and out of light hypnosis several times a day quite naturally and automatically, so there is really nothing sinister about the sensation. All the hypnotherapist does is help you achieve a trance-like state on purpose rather than leaving it to chance. No hypnotherapist can hypnotize you against your will. If you do not want to follow his or her instructions, there is nothing he or she can do.

When you are in hypnosis you direct your attention inwards. Even though you are aware of where you are and who is with you, these things are no longer at the centre of your attention. Instead, you are concentrating on the suggestions the therapist is giving you, often in the form of images. While you follow these images in your mind, you can still open your eyes whenever you want, but since the therapist will suggest a calming and peaceful scenario to you, you are less likely to feel inclined to open your eyes.

In this context, the role of the therapist is to take you on a journey into hypnosis where he is the guidebook but where you are the traveller who actually walks down the road. The therapist only facilitates hypnosis; it is the client who *goes into* hypnosis. This is why many hypnotherapists will explain to their clients that all hypnosis is really self-hypnosis.

While you are in hypnosis, you will in all likelihood experience at least some of the following sensations:

- increased watering of the eyes

- fluttering eyelids

- slower breathing

- stomach noises

- pleasant tingling in your arms and/or legs

- particular heaviness/lightness and relaxation

- feeling as if your hands/arms/legs were 'not there'

- feeling that you have become one with the chair you are sitting on

- reluctance to move

- time distortion – you will, when you are out of the hypnotic state, considerably underestimate the amount of time that you spent in hypnosis.

When coming out of hypnosis, many people feel as if they have been asleep, but they know they have not. In other words, hypnosis is a very pleasant, relaxing state to be in, where your concentration is directed inwards on to mental images – it is a bit like television in your mind! At the same time, you can expect to feel comfortably detached from the everyday world. Hypnosis is really only a shift of consciousness where inner imagery comes more to the fore and everyday reality is relegated to the back of your mind.

DIFFERENT WAYS OF USING HYPNOSIS

If you ask people in the street what they know about hypnosis, some will answer that they have seen a hypnotist on television and think it is either absolutely amazing or one big confidence trick, whereas others may know of someone who has been to see a hypnotherapist and stopped smoking/over-eating/etc. as a result.

However, there is more to hypnosis than a few suggestions to a subject on stage in order to entertain a crowd of people, and there is certainly a lot more to hypnotherapy than just quit-smoking sessions. We will now take a look at the various ways in which hypnosis can be used, both in and outside a thera-peutic context.

Under each section you will find a brief definition as well as a list of problem areas for which the particular hypnotherapy method is employed. This list of application areas should be taken as a general guideline only. You will, for example, find 'weight control' under both suggestion and analytical therapy. The reason for this is that one hypnotherapist may come from a school of thought which holds that all weight problems should be dealt with by suggestion therapy, whereas another therapist might consider suggestions insufficient and may want to find out *why* the client overeats in order to help solve the problem.

SUGGESTION THERAPY

The main application areas for suggestion therapy are:

- asthma

- bed-wetting

- childbirth

- lack of confidence

- enhancing creativity

- exam/test nerves
- hair-pulling
- improving athletic performance
- insomnia
- motivation
- nail-biting
- pain control
- sexual problems
- smoking
- stress reduction
- teeth-grinding
- ulcers
- weight control

As its name suggests, in suggestion therapy the hypnotherapist will give suggestions to the client in order to help him or her change a particular behaviour or reaction. While in hypnosis, suggestions are more easily accepted because the critical faculties of the conscious mind are partially suspended. Imagine that the conscious mind is a watchdog in front of the gates to the subconscious; by helping someone into hypnosis the watchdog is calmed down so it goes and lies down to doze while the therapist goes quietly past it and delivers positive suggestions to the subconscious mind for storage.

Once the 'goods' have been delivered to the subconscious, the client will display the desired behaviour or reaction to a greater or lesser extent once out of hypnosis. Much will depend on the quality of the suggestions given and on the rapport between therapist and client. Giving suggestions is a bit like re-recording over an old cassette tape, replacing the old message with a more positive one. Every time you start the tape from now on, it will play this new message. Instead of thinking, 'I *need* a cigarette, I'm so stressed!', you now think, 'I enjoy feeling cool, clean air flowing through my lungs, and this really relaxes me.' Instead of getting stressed when you are overloaded with work, you now think, 'I can do this!', and stay calm as you tackle the various tasks one by one.

The therapist can give you suggestions in word form or in picture form. Here are some examples:

Nail-biting

word form 'You stay calm and relaxed as you allow your fingernails to grow to their ideal length.'

picture form 'Imagine looking at your hands and seeing your nails beautifully manicured and just the right length.'

Smoking

word form 'You are a non-smoker from now on, and it is easy.'

picture form 'Imagine you could look into your body and see your lungs, coated with tar. With every day that you are a non-smoker, you can watch more and more pink patches appear.'

Weight

word form 'You find that your appetite is getting smaller and smaller and you are satisfied with far less food than you used to eat.'

picture form 'Imagine yourself in front of a full-length mirror in an outfit that is a whole size smaller, and it fits you perfectly!'

Most therapists use a mixture of both words and pictures when they give suggestions. Words are very useful because they can act as a key phrase which comes back to you throughout the day, whenever you find yourself in the previously problematic situation. You can even repeat the key phrase ('I can do this!'; 'I am calm and relaxed') consciously like a positive affirmation to further deepen the effectiveness of the post-hypnotic suggestion.

Pictures, on the other hand, have a more three-dimensional quality to them. For many people the image of, for example, themselves in front of a mirror having reached their desired size triggers positive feelings much more readily than the words 'I lose weight easily and effortlessly.' This is possibly because, in some respects, the subconscious mind is like a six-year-old – it loves cartoons! So if you give it pictures as well as words, it acts upon them even more enthusiastically.

Some people are worried that they will be unable to see pictures in their minds and therefore will not gain the full benefit of suggestion therapy; they feel they have no imagination. But this is no stumbling block in hypnotherapy.

To visualize means to see something in your mind's eye, and we all visualize quite naturally every day. Whenever someone asks us directions, we have to reconstruct the route in our minds. Whenever we listen to someone else describing their holidays, and even when we read a novel, we automatically produce pictures in our minds. Remember the last time you went to see a film *after* you had read the book on which it was based? You were probably disappointed because the characters in the film *did not look like you imagined them when you read the book*.

Seeing an image in your mind is, for most people, much more vague than seeing with your eyes open; it is more like having an idea of what something looks like rather than having a sharply defined picture in your mind. As long as you can roughly describe to someone else what you have imagined, your visualization skills are good enough for hypnotherapy.

But what about suggestibility? Can anyone be hypnotized, and what are the characteristics that make a person a good hypnotic subject? Researchers in the US, Canada, Australia and Germany have come to very similar conclusions about this. About 10 per cent of people are very susceptible to hypnosis, 10 per cent are very difficult to hypnotize, and the other 80 per cent are somewhere in between and make reasonably good hypnotic subjects.

It is often wrongly assumed that only weak-willed or very gullible people can be hypnotized. This is not so. It is those who are reasonably intelligent, creative and imaginative people who are good subjects, with children being among the best. People who are difficult to hypnotize are either of very limited intelligence or have a great fear of losing control, as are people who have difficulty really enjoying themselves.

Here is a questionnaire which will help you decide whether you are among the 90 per cent of people who can be hypnotized well. Answer 'yes' or 'no' to every statement; give yourself 1 point for every 'yes'.

1. Have you in the past or do you now practise relaxation such as yoga or meditation with good results?

2. Do you have artistic inclinations and/or talents?

3. Can you get so involved in an activity that you forget the time?

4. Can you get wrapped up in your thoughts so that you are 'miles away' in your mind?

5. When you watch a good film in the cinema, are you so captivated that, at times, you feel you are in the film?

6. Do pleasant memories create pleasant sensations in you?

7. Do unpleasant memories make you feel uncomfortable?

8. Do you have a vivid imagination?

9. Do you express your feelings easily?

10. Are there people whom you trust completely?

0 – 2 points	*You are not easy to hypnotize.*
3 – 8 points	*You are among the 80 per cent of people who are of average-to-good suggestibility.*
9 – 10 points	*You are a hypnotherapist's dream!*

Suggestion therapy is a very effective tool for many conditions such as negative habits and low performance levels, and, provided the client is reasonably suggestible (it is not necessary to be in the top 10 per cent), between one and three sessions should help solve the problem. In this context, it does not even matter whether you believe that hypnotherapy will work for you. There are many seasoned smokers on 60 to 100 cigarettes a day who have doubted very much that they could give up the habit after 30 years of uninterrupted smoking, only to find, when trying hypnotherapy as a last resort, that in spite of their scepticism they are in fact able to stop smoking . . .

There are circumstances, however, under which suggestions may not work for you. Sometimes a habit problem is masking a much more deep-rooted difficulty. A client may come for weight control treatment when the real problem is anxiety; or a client in a creative profession who is experiencing a block may not respond to positive suggestions because the block is an accumulation of various traumatic incidents that have happened in the past, triggered by something in the present that has reactivated the negative feelings to do with the past trauma. In these cases, analytical hypnotherapy is needed to remove the underlying cause so that the symptoms disappear as well. More of this in a later section (*see page 27*).

Another reason why suggestions might not take hold is that the client may derive a secondary gain from a problem. A woman may come for therapy to get rid of tension headaches but may find she gets no relief through the treatment. On closer inspection it could turn out that the only times her family are kind and considerate to her is when she is feeling unwell, so by hanging on to her symptoms she ensures that she is not missing out on much-needed attention which she feels she cannot get any other way. In such a case, the obvious course of action is to help the client build up her confidence so that she can ask her family for attention in a more constructive way.

What can also prevent suggestions from taking root in the subconscious is if you dislike or mistrust the hypnotherapist. If you feel uncomfortable in the therapist's presence, you will be less likely to relax or go along with the suggestions. Also, if the suggestions are against your moral beliefs or do not make sense to you, you will simply reject them. This is why it is important for the therapist to ask you in detail about what the problem is, so that the suggestions can be tailormade to your particular case. Remember – you cannot be hypnotized against your will, and you will also not accept suggestions that you disagree with.

DESENSITIZATION THERAPY

Desensitization therapy shares quite a few aspects with general suggestion therapy; however, there are sufficient differences to warrant its own section here.

Desensitization means approaching a fear-inducing situation

or object step by step until that situation or object no longer creates fear in the subject. Each step is first practised mentally in hypnosis, then, when clients feel comfortable with the mental process, they are encouraged to test it in reality.

Fears and phobias are the main application area for desensitization. Here are a few examples, but please be aware that this list is far from being complete.

Desensitization can help with fear of:

- an animal or insect (spiders, mice, snakes, worms, cats, dogs, birds, etc.)

- being alone

- crossing bridges

- crowds

- darkness

- eating in public

- enclosed spaces (lifts, underground trains, flying in a plane)

- heights

- illness

- water.

Desensitization is used with fears and phobias in both therapist-directed hypnotherapy and self-hypnosis. A phobia can be distinguished from an ordinary fear by three factors:

a)   it is persistent over a long period;

b) the fear is clearly unreasonable but sufferers cannot stop themselves from feeling afraid;

c) sufferers tend to try and avoid the fear-inducing object or situation.

Not all fears and phobias will require desensitization; in cases where the fear is not too strong or has not existed for too long, the hypnotherapist may very well be able to use straightforward suggestion therapy. Some therapists will always start with suggestion therapy, no matter how severe the fear, and move on to gradual desensitization or analytical hypnotherapy only if the fear does not respond to suggestion therapy.

When desensitization is used, the therapist will first of all ensure that you can experience good physical relaxation while in hypnosis, and may well spend a session or two on this. As fears and phobias are often induced by stress, the fact that you can generally stay calmer and more relaxed will already take the edge off your fear. The next task is to find out what the steps are that can take you to your goal of encountering the difficult situation or object without fear. Let us look at an example of fear of lifts, and let us assume that your fear is so great that you have been avoiding lifts altogether for the last year. Your aim would obviously be to get into a lift and stay calm and relaxed, no matter how many floors up or down you were travelling.

Your therapist would first of all start by segmenting the achievement of your aim into smaller and more manageable pieces. The segmentation could look as follows:

1. standing by a lift door, watching the doors open and close while people use it and staying calm and relaxed all the while

2. pressing the button to call the lift and watching the doors open and close again while still remaining outside

3. calling the lift by pressing the button, stepping inside, remaining there for a few moments with your finger on the 'door open' button, then stepping out of the lift again

4. calling the lift, stepping inside, allowing the doors to close and going up or down one floor.

Once the therapist has helped you into a comfortable state of hypnotic relaxation, he or she will talk you through the first step, describing for you the experience of standing by the side of the lift and watching other people use it. The therapist might have agreed a signal with you, such as the raising of a finger, so you can tell him or her if you are feeling uncomfortable at any stage. If you begin to feel tense as a step is being described to you, the therapist will go back a step. If you feel OK with the first step, the therapist will ask you to test this against reality, suggesting that you soon try standing next to a real lift.

In cases where clients cannot even think about the phobia-inducing situation or object without getting tense, a therapist might ask them to put the object of their fear on to a screen in their minds so that they can detach themselves more from the object and stay calmer.

Some people are so scared of, for example, snakes or worms that they cannot even look at a photograph of one without getting upset or panicky. In these cases the therapist might suggest that they imagine the snake or worm as a cartoon with a silly hat and glasses on.

In addition to the work that is being done in the sessions, a therapist may also give clients a self-hypnosis tape for general relaxation; this becomes their 'homework' for the duration of treatment. The tape helps to get clients' overall stress levels down and makes them stay calm and feel more in control, and thus diminishes their feelings of fear.

To sum up, in the desensitization process it is important to start with the smallest possible step that will allow the client to stay calm and relaxed while experiencing that step in hypnosis. The therapist will then slowly build up the client's confidence by gradually introducing more and more advanced steps until the target – experiencing the real-life situation without fear – is reached.

ANALYTICAL HYPNOTHERAPY

This form of hypnotherapy is also know as hypno-analysis. Its objective is to discover the underlying reason for a presenting symptom and, by working through the cause, making the symptom redundant.

The main application areas for analytical hypnotherapy are:

- addictive behaviour
- anxiety
- asthma
- depression
- eating disorders (bingeing, anorexia, bulimia)
- eczema
- lack of confidence
- lack of self-worth
- obsessions and compulsions
- panic attacks
- phobias

- psoriasis
- sexual problems
- weight control

Let us look at an example to illustrate the workings of analytical hypnotherapy.

Anna, a young woman of 24, had been suffering from low self-esteem ever since she could remember. She put herself down whenever she was in company and she expected to fail at whatever she attempted. She decided to go for therapy when she found she had scared away a nice man who had shown an interest in her, simply because she did not believe she deserved him. She realized she had alienated him by her rude and abrupt behaviour, and now wanted to sort out her problem in the hopes of avoiding a repetition of the same mistake with a potential new boyfriend.

In her hypnotherapy sessions with me, I helped Anna explore her feelings of worthlessness and to trace them back in time to where they originally came from. Anna remembered feeling incompetent and foolish in secondary school, where she had been picked on by a teacher who took pleasure in humiliating her in front of everybody. But this had not been the first time that Anna had been given to understand that she was useless. When Anna traced her feelings of worthlessness and rejection further back, she remembered her father being very critical of her and never praising her when she had achieved something, whereas her brother could do no wrong. Anna's mother, a quiet and withdrawn woman, was no help either; she kept out of things and never defended her daughter against the father. When things started going wrong at school and the teacher began bullying Anna, she felt she had no one to turn to. Her mother was not interested and her father just waved Anna away, telling her that she must have done something to deserve the teacher's scorn.

During her sessions I helped Anna deal with the memories of the teacher, her mother and her father so that all her pent-up emotions of despair, hopelessness and anger could be vented and linked up with the original memories where they belonged. Anna realized that she was not at all a useless person but that others had treated her as such. She was now able to step back from her father's criticism and regard his harsh judgement of her as an opinion which she, Anna, did not share any longer. She gained in confidence considerably, even while she was still attending hypnotherapy, and left after ten sessions a much happier and more confident person. She went on to apply for a new, better paid job and eventually got married to a lovely man whom she now felt she deserved.

I used a technique called *regression* with Anna, as you have seen. Regression entails asking clients to take a feeling they are experiencing at the moment and trace this feeling back to where it occurred before. This will often lead all the way back into childhood. As children we are particularly receptive to what adults say to us or about us. If we are exposed to a great deal of negative feedback about our person, this affects our self-image adversely and forms a pattern for our adult thinking about ourselves and others. In Anna's case, she had learned through her parents' and teacher's behaviour that she was inadequate and unimportant, and that even when she genuinely needed help she would not get it at home. Anna then went on to live her life accordingly – before anyone else could find out how worthless she was, she would pre-empt them and say so herself; if others were nice to her, she thought they were either lying and just trying to be polite, or that they were too stupid to see that she was not worth their attention. Her consequent rudeness was only natural, because she felt that people who were nice to her were either condescending or irritating in their stupidity.

Analytical hypnotherapy is centred around the client's memories and consequently requires the client to speak during hypnosis. While you are in hypnosis, your concentration is better and your powers of recall are much enhanced so that it becomes easier to access events that have happened in the past. In some people, the ease with which they recollect early childhood events in great detail can be quite stunning – they remember the pattern of the wallpaper when they were in their playpen, and even have memories of when they were lying in their cot! However, not everyone has such detailed and vivid recollections from their earliest years. Luckily, that does not really matter because everyone has direct or indirect access to at least a few relevant memories.

Sometimes memories can be suppressed because the initial event was so traumatic at the time that the only way for the client to have stayed intact as a person was to hide the memory away. This repression can happen if you witness or are involved in a violent incident or a tragic accident; it can also happen if you have been the victim of sexual abuse. Please note that repression of such memories is not *automatic*, but it *can* occur in some people. If this is the case, hypnosis can help reveal the original trauma and bring it to the surface so that the client can be helped to work through it and get over it. As long as a traumatic event stays hidden, it has power over you because it can produce symptoms such as depression, self-hatred, anxiety and the like.

Over the years there have been lots of discussions about the topic of analysis versus suggestion therapy. It has been said that it might be dangerous to look at hidden memories because they have been hidden for a good reason and therefore should not be meddled with. This objection to analysis is certainly justified if the therapist allows clients to re-experience the trauma and then does not help them to work through it. If clients are just left with the difficult memory, the therapist is irresponsible. Any well-trained hypno-analyst will know that it is essential to support the client if such a memory resurfaces.

The fact is, however, that most clients undergoing analytical hypnotherapy will not have any such major repressed memories. The majority of clients will remember things in hypnosis that they knew about anyway, with one significant difference: they have forgotten how much this past situation affected them at the time.

Here are examples of past events that often lay at the bottom of present-day problems:

- one or both parents being over-critical

- one or both parents ignoring you

- being bullied at school by classmates or teachers

- having other siblings preferred over you

- feeling 'different' as a child because
  –you have no father/mother
  –you come from a different social class to your classmates (richer *or* poorer)
  –you have a physical disability

- emotional cruelty/blackmail by people you depend on

- guilt about a mistake you once made

- having been involved in a very embarrassing situation

- physical/sexual abuse.

Re-experiencing past trauma in hypnosis helps release pent-up emotions and enables the client to let go of the past. Sometimes this process (known as *abreaction*) can take the form of a tearful outburst; sometimes it can be a very quiet matter where clients suddenly realize that something that happened in the past was not their fault after all, and this realization is coupled with a great sense of relief.

Hypnosis is an invaluable tool in facilitating memory recall, but it is not a truth-drug that will make you say things you do not want to speak about. It is perfectly possible for a client to withhold information while in hypnosis. Sometimes an embarrassing memory might come up and the client may feel reluctant to talk about it and decide not to mention it. Therapists will usually point out to clients in the initial consultation that such a situation might arise, and will try to encourage clients to overcome this resistance. Any resistance is a sign that a particular past event constitutes some unfinished emotional business.

There are two different ways of experiencing the process of recall in hypnosis. Clients who are among the top ten per cent of extremely suggestible personalities (*see page 18*) will feel as if they are 'in' the memory. If they go back to the age of five, they start speaking in a child's tone of voice and use very simple vocabulary, just as a little child would. The majority of people, however, will only partially regress, which means that although they are recalling past events, they are aware that they are only talking about a memory; in other words, they think on two levels – while they remember, they still hold on to the present. Whether people regress totally or only partially, they can still get the same good results from the analytical hypnotherapy process. The depth of hypnosis a person is capable of depends on each individual's disposition; luckily the positive outcome of hypnotherapy is not dependent on the depth of hypnosis a person can achieve.

SELF-HYPNOSIS

In self-hypnosis you become your own therapist and use the power of your subconscious mind to influence a particular habit or behaviour. Main application areas for self-hypnosis are:

- accelerating learning
- accelerating recovery after illness
- building self-confidence
- enhancing creativity
- exam/test nerves
- hair-pulling
- improving performance
- nailbiting
- pain control
- skin-picking
- sleeping problems
- smoking
- tension headaches
- weight control.

Self-hypnosis is ideal for helping yourself overcome any of the above problems. People are often prescribed tranquillizers, painkillers or beta blockers for some of these conditions, yet you can get very good results by using hypnosis, with the added advantage that it is pleasant, non-toxic and often much more effective than tablets. If you have any of the problems mentioned above, provided there are no serious emotional causes underlying these problems you can learn to use self-hypnosis to store positive suggestions in your subconscious and help yourself.

In order to use self-hypnosis successfully you will have to learn a few techniques and stick to some simple rules.

SETTING AN AIM

Be specific about what you want. Without a clear aim you will find it difficult to select the right suggestions and images.

–If you want to lose weight, how much do you want to lose?

–If you want to cut down on smoking, how many cigarettes do you want to cut down to?

–If you want to be more confident, which situation do you want to cope with better?

Set yourself a clear aim and tackle only one aim at a time. You may want to improve your tennis, lose half a stone in weight and have a better memory, but do not try and do all three at once. Pick the goal which, for whatever reason, is most important to you right now; tackle other issues later.

WRITING A SCRIPT

The next step is to put together a number of suggestions which will help you reach your chosen aim. Here are some examples:

Driving Test Nerves
Your aim is to pass your driving test and stay calm and relaxed during the test.

I am calm and relaxed, my breathing is regular and even. I am well prepared and I have successfully practised driving during my lessons. Everything is fine. I am ready and comfortable to demonstrate my skills in the driving test. I am calm and collected as I get into the car to start the test; everything is running smoothly and easily. I'm calm and concentrated; everything is going well. I remember all the rules easily and effortlessly and drive carefully and competently. I breathe easily, my movements are smooth and confident, my mind is easy and free. At the end of the test, both my examiner and my instructor congratulate me on my excellent performance.

Losing Weight
Your aim is to lose five pounds.

I am now ready to let go of the excess pounds which I no longer need or want. I'm letting go of the extra weight easily and effortlessly. My appetite is getting smaller and smaller; it is as if my stomach has shrunk a little and simply cannot take in as much food as it used to. I feel lighter and freer with every day, losing the excess pounds one by one, and it is so easy! I eat modest portions of good food, and I am satisfied, completely satisfied, and I can already see myself in front of a full-length mirror, wearing those jeans/that skirt/outfit [choose something you can only get into once you have lost the weight] and it fits me perfectly. I look great and I feel great, light and free.

Improving Confidence
Your aim is to become more confident in work meetings.

As I'm going into the meeting, I am calm and relaxed. I am aware that I know most of the people there and that makes me feel really comfortable. I have a brief, relaxed chat with the person sitting next to me at the conference table as I settle back comfortably. I am calm, and concentrate on what is being said by others. I listen attentively and get deeply involved in the issues raised. I am well prepared and I have something to say which is helpful and of importance to the meeting. I feel good about myself and I feel good within myself, and I speak easily and fluently, my breathing is regular and even and my movements are free and easy. I am speaking clearly and people listen attentively. I am so involved in what is going on in the meeting that I get carried along with it easily and effortlessly. I contribute to the meeting confidently and in a professional manner, and at the end of the meeting I feel pleased that I have done so well.

Looking at these three examples, you may have already noticed that they have a few things in common. These are the rules that you should observe when writing a script:

USE POSITIVE WORDING

The subconscious mind tends to take suggestions literally, so you would do best to avoid negative phrasing.

Not 'I will not be afraid' *but* 'I feel confident.'
Not 'I stop feeling stressed' *but* 'I am calm and relaxed.'
Not 'I must not overeat' *but* 'I eat modest portions.'

Say what you want, not what you don't want.

USE THE PRESENT TENSE

If you word a suggestion by using the future tense, your subconscious mind can end up waiting with you for this positive event to happen, rather than getting on with it now. Although it is not always possible to phrase your suggestion in the present tense, you should try to do so wherever possible.

Not 'I will be more confident' *but* 'I am more confident with every day that passes by.'

Not 'I will speak fluently at the conference' *but* 'I am calm and relaxed and speak confidently.'

However, some phrases only exist in the future tense. If you are having problems sleeping at night, the suggestion 'Everything will be all right' is very useful. It has a soothing effect and is a simple childlike way to reassure and relax your body and mind.

REPEAT SUGGESTIONS

When you construct a script, say the same thing repeatedly, using different words where possible to make it more interesting. Here are some examples.

'I am calm and relaxed. I feel comfortable, and a lovely sense of tranquillity spreads through my body and mind. I enjoy the serene and calm feeling inside.'

'I am drifting off into sound sleep. I can feel myself getting sleepier and sleepier, as thoughts of the day drift away gently. My body relaxes and my mind slows down.'

Even if you cannot rephrase something by putting it into different words, do not worry. Just use the same phrase repeatedly throughout the script.

USE EMOTIVE WORDS

The more positive emotions your script evokes, the more readily your subconscious mind will convert the suggestions into action. Be generous with terms like 'wonderful', 'deep', 'complete' or 'excellent'. 'I feel deeply relaxed,' for example, is more powerful than 'I feel relaxed;' 'I am completely at ease' is better than 'I am at ease.'

MAKE IT PERFECT

Do not be half-hearted about your script and do not build in any flaws to make it more realistic. A script is not about reality, it is about raising positive expectations and thereby creating a relaxed but concentrated frame of mind. When you are relaxed you are much more efficient when you need to sort out a problem should it arise, so make sure your script helps you to be poised and confident; the rest will follow naturally.

PREPARE WELL

The best script for exam nerves will not do a thing for you unless you have prepared for the exam. No script in the world will help you pass a test, or lose weight, or achieve any other goal if you have not laid the groundwork first.

USE IMAGES

Whenever possible include a picture in your script. You may have noticed that in the examples on losing weight and passing the driving test, images were used to give the script more depth and make it more three-dimensional ('I can already see myself in front of a full-length mirror;' 'I am calm and collected as I get into the car to start the test').

Now you know how to write a script, you will need to learn how to go into and come out of hypnosis. Here is an easy exercise to get you started. Read through the following three sections first before you try them out.

Fractional Induction

- Make yourself comfortable, sitting or lying down. Loosen any tight clothing.

- Close your eyes. Sit still for a moment so that you can become aware of how you are sitting in the chair or lying on the bed. Be aware of where your head is, your shoulders, arms and hands, your back, your legs and feet. Do not move; just *think* about the different parts of your body.

- Start off by tensing the muscles in your feet. Hold the tension, feel the tension, then *slowly* let the tension go. While you are doing this, imagine what your feet look like as they tense up and what they look like as they relax again.

- Continue the tensing and relaxing as follows: calf muscles, thighs, belly area, chest area, hands and arms together, shoulders, jaw muscles, forehead.

This induction method will help you relax your body and concentrate your mind, so that you are now already in very light hypnosis and receptive to suggestions. Now go on to the next step and deepen the hypnosis a little more.

Counting Down

In your mind, count down from ten to zero. While you are doing this, imagine that you are going down the steps of a beautiful staircase. With every step downward you go deeper into hypnosis, getting more and more relaxed. At the bottom of the steps you find a door that leads into a beautiful room. As your hand touches the doorknob, you are even more deeply relaxed. Enter the room and find a comfortable chair. Sit down and, as you are sinking back into the chair, you go to your deepest level of relaxation. Imagine this room to be the centre of your mind where there is always peace and harmony, and where all things are possible.

Counting Up

Whenever you want to come out of hypnosis, simply leave your room again and start walking up the steps, counting in your mind from one to ten. When you are at the top of the steps, on the count of ten, open your eyes again and think the words 'wide awake'.

Practise the fractional induction, counting down and then counting up again a few times; then add your script when you have counted yourself down and are in the comfortable chair in your beautiful room. The easiest way to do this is by speaking everything on to a cassette tape and then listening to the tape through headphones – a simple Walkman will work very well. If you do not have a tape recorder, memorize a few key sentences from your script, ideally coupled to a positive image of having achieved your aim, and use this remembered material after counting down.

WARNING: If you make a tape, never use it while driving or operating machinery. As self-hypnosis can be extremely relaxing, you could have an accident if you are doing anything else while listening to the tape.

When you are using self-hypnosis you do not have to go into a deep trance to get results. Even if you can get just a little bit relaxed and concentrated you will be able to improve on your chosen area, provided you use your self-hypnosis script regularly (at least once a day) for a minimum of three weeks. Remember that your subconscious mind has been used to reacting in one particular way, often over a period of many years, so it will take a persistent and repeated effort to 'reprogramme' it.

If you feel you are unable to put all this practice in, you may prefer to go to a hypnotherapist for some sessions of suggestion therapy.

STAGE HYPNOSIS

Even though stage hypnosis is not used in a therapeutic context, it is still included in this book because many of the myths and misunderstandings that exist about hypnosis arise from the not-always-ethical performances on stage and television. Members of the audience are often not sure whether what they are seeing is a trick, with subjects just pretending that they are in hypnosis, or whether the hypnotist has some supernatural powers that he can use to make people do what he wants them to do.

Some critics say that anything you can do in hypnosis you can do without hypnosis anyway. They claim that anyone can pretend to sing like Elvis Presley or pretend to be stiff as a board so that he or she can be suspended between two chairs. This may be true for a lot of the tasks hypnotists give their subjects on stage, but it is not the whole story. What about eating an onion without your eyes watering? You can in hypnosis, but you cannot in a non-hypnotic state. What about a haemophiliac in hypnosis undergoing dental surgery without losing blood? Hardly something that we can all do anyway ...

You have already read in previous chapters that there is nothing mysterious about hypnosis and that most people can go at least into a light trance. But these are not the people a stage hypnotist wants for a show; he wants people who come into the 10 per cent bracket of highly suggestible types. Hypnotic shows therefore usually take place in an environment such as a festival hall, a big party or a nightclub where a great number of people are present. The more people, the greater the likelihood to find those who are easy to hypnotize.

When the hypnotist comes on stage he will often start with a general explanation of hypnosis; in doing so he will already be giving out hidden suggestions by emphasizing words such as 'relaxing' and 'enjoyable' and repeating them a lot, usually quite inconspicuously. Good hypnotic subjects will already feel a bit more relaxed and will start sinking comfortably back into their seats . . . The hypnotist then continues with some openly announced experiments or tests, asking people in the audience to clasp their hands in front of them, fingers interlaced, and then suggesting that 'your fingers feel like they are glued together and no matter how hard you try, you cannot take your hands apart.' At this point at least half the audience will think, 'Of course I can!' and just take their hands apart, while another percentage of the audience will be a bit unsure but will then try and succeed in disengaging their fingers. This leaves the rest, who sit there and simply cannot get their hands apart. The hypnotist will then announce that now, everyone can feel their hands coming unstuck, and with a sigh of relief this last group will feel they can let their hands come apart.

Some similar tests might follow, and then those people who responded positively to the tests are asked to come forward. Now the hypnotist can 'prime' these very suggestible subjects by putting them into hypnosis and giving them a post-hypnotic suggestion – such as that whenever he snaps his fingers they will go into deep hypnosis. Now he can go ahead and give them more suggestions to elicit all sorts of peculiar and amusing behaviour. However, please remember that if he tried to do this with anyone else in the audience, he could not do it.

On television you are not usually shown the initial selection process, so you are left with the impression that some amazing powers are at work. All you see is the hypnotist snapping his fingers and the subjects doing as they are told. No wonder so many people are still frightened of going to a hypnotherapist!

The problem with stage hypnosis lies in the fact that the hypnotist does not know anything at all about the people who come on stage. All he knows is that they are highly suggestible. He does not know whether they have any serious emotional problems which could be exacerbated if they were asked to go back to their childhood. Nor does he know if they have any medical problems that might make them unfit for any strenuous exercise or some of the tasks he may ask them to perform.

There is still very little criminal law specifically relating to stage hypnosis. The British Hypnotism Act dates back to 1952

40

and states that demonstrations of hypnotism should be limited to places that are licensed for public entertainment, and that it is unlawful to hypnotize someone on stage who is under 21 years of age. These conditions are of course far from sufficient to protect the public from unethical hypnotists, and ultimately the greatest safety lies in ensuring that the hypnotist is also a qualified and practising hypnotherapist who chooses the stage act carefully and is able to handle any unexpected reactions the subjects may experience.

CAUTIONS AND CONTRA-INDICATIONS

There are a few circumstances in which hypnosis should not be used.

In cases where a person suffers from epilepsy, hypnosis is not indicated as it could trigger an epileptic fit.

Another area where hypnotherapy cannot help is in cases where a person suffers from a psychosis rather than a neurosis. The main difference between a neurosis and a psychosis is that sufferers with a neurotic disorder are aware that they have a problem; they can recognize that their fears are either irrational or exaggerated. Those afflicted with a psychosis, on the other hand, are convinced that they are normal in their fears and that it is others who are thoughtlessly unaware of the dangers that they perceive as very real.

In the context of hypnotherapy this means that a hypnotherapist would be unable to help anyone who suffers from illusions or delusions or any form of schizophrenia.

YOUR QUESTIONS ANSWERED

Can everybody be hypnotized?
Nearly everybody. The exceptions are people who are drunk

PRINCIPLES OF HYPNOTHERAPY

Will my mind be interfered with?

No. If the therapist suggests something to you that is against your moral beliefs, you will simply not carry out the suggestion.

Will I change personality?

No. What hypnotherapy does is to help bring out the best in you. This means that you will change by leaving behind any habits or emotional baggage you no longer need or want and thereby become a stronger and happier person. Hypnosis will not put something into you that was not there in the first place; it just helps you to uncover your strong and good qualities which you may not even have known you had.

Will I remember what happens during the sessions?

Ninety-nine per cent of people do remember everything they or the therapist said during the session. In rare instances clients might not remember, but if the therapist reminds them of one or two points that were talked about, they tend to remember the whole session. It is also possible for a therapist to give a post-hypnotic suggestion for the client to forget what was said, but this is rarely done in a therapeutic context.

Will the therapist have to touch me?

Some therapists will lay a hand on your shoulder or on your arm, others might lift up your hand or lightly move your head to test whether you are properly relaxed. There are also therapists who put a finger on your forehead to induce hypnosis. Other than this form of contact, a therapist has no business touching you. The vast majority of therapists are ethical, and transgressions are rare, but should you experience any unwanted physical contact you may want to get in touch with the professional body your therapist is a member of and report the matter.

HOW HYPNOTHERAPY
CAN HELP

Many people believe or are told that they have to learn to live with their depression, anxiety or panic attacks, but luckily this is not so. There are a great number of problem areas and symptoms that hypnotherapy can help effectively and relatively quickly, provided you see a well-qualified and experienced hypnotherapist.

There is no symptom without a cause. If you feel anxious or if you lack confidence there is a reason for it, even though you may not be aware of that reason. A symptom is always a warning signal which tells you that something is wrong. Physical pain urges you to look at what is happening with your body; psychological distress is a sign that you need to attend to some emotional matter. Just as physical pain can be switched off by painkillers, emotional pain can be numbed by taking tranquillizers. However, taking tablets can never be a permanent solution. Anti-depressants, tranquillizers and beta blockers are acceptable for a short period, but if the problem has not righted itself after six months it will be necessary to look for the underlying cause. Taking tablets will take the edge off a symptom but they do not remove the cause; all you are doing is wallpapering over the cracks. Many problems go away by themselves, and many can be overcome by applying common-sense self-help techniques. If, however, a psychological diffi-culty persists, you should seek professional help.

If a problem is stress-induced, suggestion hypnotherapy can help reduce the stress and thereby make the symptom super-fluous. With habits such as smoking or nailbiting, reducing stress and planting positive suggestions in the subconscious mind is usually enough to overcome the habit. With more com-plex problems such as anxiety and depression, a more detailed approach needs to be taken to reveal and work through the underlying cause.

HABITS

Habits can be very tenacious once they have become estab-lished. Among the most common habits people come to a hyp-notherapist for are the following:

- smoking

- nail-biting

- hair-pulling

- skin-picking

- thumb-sucking

- teeth-grinding.

Just as we can learn to shift the gear lever automatically as we drive a car, without having to think about it, we can become accustomed to pulling our hair or lighting a cigarette, only half aware that we are doing so. Sometimes it is only at the end of the day when you notice the empty packet that you become aware of how many cigarettes you have smoked during the day.

Alternatively, you may *know* you are performing a certain habit but cannot stop yourself. It is as if you have two parts within you: one part knows all the logical reasons why you should not go ahead and give in to your habit yet again, but the other part just runs away with you and does it anyway. Then follows an inner stream of recriminations and annoyance at being so weak-willed, which in turn makes you feel stressed and consequently provokes another spree of smoking, hair-pulling or nail-biting. It is a vicious circle.

In order to help a client leave a habit behind, it is important for the therapist to find out about the hidden emotional benefits of that habit and the client's motivation to stop. Even though some habits are clearly unhealthy (smoking) or disfiguring (hair-pulling, nail-biting), they nevertheless serve a purpose for the individual. Often a sense of comfort is derived from the habit, and sometimes the habit operates as a release valve when stress starts to build up. Smoking is often an excuse for taking a break or keeping your hands and mouth busy.

Reasons for wanting to break a habit will vary from person to person, although there are some general points that are mentioned by most clients:

- embarrassment about the habit

- social unacceptability

- vanity (smoking ages the skin prematurely; hair-pulling thins out one's hair, skin-picking disfigures the skin)

- health reasons (smoking causes cancer; grinding the teeth wears them down and damages the gums).

As the therapist finds out about clients' perception of the benefits of their habit and their motivation for stopping, these details can be integrated into the hypnotic suggestions. That way, each session is individually tailormade and therefore more likely to get good results.

This type of suggestion therapy can take anything between one and five sessions. If no improvement occurs after two sessions it is usually recommended that client and hypnotherapist together start to deal with the reasons why the client cannot let go of the habit. This might take the form of so-called pinpoint analysis, where the therapist helps the client find the reason for the inner blockage. Pinpoint analysis usually takes one or two sessions and deals only with feelings and memories related directly to the habit. The client is then helped to see the relevant past event in a different light so that it need not obstruct progress in overcoming the habit any longer.

The following two case histories show one straightforward session of suggestion therapy and one where pinpoint analysis had to be used. In all the case histories in this book the names of clients have been changed to ensure confidentiality.

Case History: Smoking (1)

Gerald (62) was a businessman whose background was that of public school, RAF and later as a commercial airline pilot. He had been smoking since the age of 16 and was on 80 cigarettes a day when he came for treatment. His doctor had told him to stop smoking, but no one in his family, including himself, believed he could do it. Because he felt so hopeless about giving up I decided to look for an earlier event in his life which had presented him with problems and which he had subsequently conquered. Luckily, it turned out that just such an example existed.

When Gerald changed from the RAF to commercial piloting he had to start from scratch. Even though he had held a high rank in the airforce he was forced to start again as a low-ranking officer, having to take orders from people far less experienced than himself. He admitted that this had been a trying time for him initially, but ultimately he had managed to work himself up to a good position again. I asked him how he had managed to get through that unpleasant initial period, and his answer was, 'Oh well, I just got on with it!'

I consequently included this phrase in the hypnotic suggestions, implying that, just like way back then, he might occasionally feel it was a bit difficult to be a non-smoker, but that if that thought came to his mind he would simply tell himself to get on with it. This suggestion was coupled with more general issues such as relaxing more, enjoying the freedom of being a non-smoker and appreciating all the positive side-effects, such as increased energy and great pride in himself.

Gerald stopped smoking after one session; a follow-up showed that he was still not smoking three years after that session.

Case History: Smoking (2)

Jane was smoking about 20 cigarettes a day when she came for treatment. She professed that she did not even like smoking, and yet she seemed unable to stop. After one session of suggestion therapy she had cut down to one cigarette a day, which she would smoke in her husband's presence. She did not understand why she felt compelled to do so. She obviously needed someone to see her being unsuccessful.

In the second session I asked Jane (while she was in hypnosis) what it might feel like if she succeeded at giving up smoking. She said it would be scary. I asked her to hang on to that scary feeling and go back in time to find where that feeling had occurred for the first time. Jane went straight back to her school days, when she had been a very diligent student who got excellent marks. While her brother and sister were out playing she sat indoors, doing her homework. Still, she had one best friend with whom she spent a lot of time at school.

One day her friend had been given the task of making sure that no one entered the school building during break, but Jane had sneaked in to retrieve something she had forgotten. Her friend saw her and reported her to a teacher, and Jane was punished. This was the end of their friendship. Jane came to believe that her friend was jealous of her studiousness and accomplishments, and concluded that others will dislike you if you are too good and too successful, and that you lose friends if they become envious of your success.

Jane had carried the same fear with her to the present day. If she stopped smoking, she would lose her friends; that was why she smoked in front of someone, to show she was not that good after all ... I asked Jane, while still in hypnosis, to put herself into the shoes of her present-day best friend and experience what it would feel like to be told that she had managed to stop smoking. Jane reported that she would be overjoyed to hear this news. After this second session, Jane was able to stop smoking altogether.

DEPRESSION AND ANXIETY

These two conditions are mentioned under the same heading because, even though they can occur on their own, they often appear together. Sometimes the depression is more prevalent, sometimes the anxiety is the dominant feature.

DEPRESSION

Among the main features of depression are:

- crying

- difficulty sleeping at night

- loss of your sense of humour

- listlessness

- negative outlook on life

- withdrawal from social life

- desire to be alone

- feelings of helplessness

- inability to cope with even minor stresses

- loss of sexual desire

- loss of appetite

- constant fatigue

- lack of concentration.

Depression can have a variety of origins. The most easily understandable type of depression comes from having suffered a traumatic loss. This could be the death of a partner, a child or even a beloved pet. Equally, being made redundant or heavy financial burdens can result in depression. On the whole, sufferers tend to come out of these depressions by themselves after sufficient time has elapsed after the triggering event. If this is not the case, professional help is needed.

Another possible cause of depression is repressed anger. If you have not been allowed to express negative emotions, or if anger was only shown in its violent form during your childhood, you may have learned to suppress and ignore it. However, life does not always run smoothly; things go wrong and people sometimes treat us disrespectfully. Without being able to feel anger and then use it constructively, we are left feeling helpless and vulnerable, and the easiest way to avoid any further unpleasant situations is to withdraw from the world.

A component of hidden anger can also play a role in postnatal depression. If you had an unhappy childhood yourself and are now confronted with your own baby whom you are supposed to love and look after, this can bring back feelings of anger at never having received the love you needed, and resentment at having to give to your child what you never had yourself.

A further factor that can lead to depression is something called learned helplessness. Being brought up in an overprotective environment where you were neither allowed nor taught to deal with the everyday world can make you feel incompetent and vulnerable when you finally leave that environment.

Case History: Depression

Paul, a young man of 24, came for treatment for a depression which he had suffered from for seven years, on and off. It had started when he first learned that his parents were going to separate.

During analytical hypnotherapy he experienced a great sense of abandonment when remembering this occasion, even though he was already 17 years old at the time. This seemed to suggest that the depressed feelings dated back to a time before his parents split up. As his earlier years of childhood started unfolding, it became clear that his father had been absent a lot and his mother was undemonstrative and incapable of showing any warmth to her children. She was preoccupied with her own life and was unable to give her three children the attention and affection they craved. In order to get any attention at all, Paul tried to be particularly good and helpful, but somehow he never managed to gain his mother's approval. When he left for boarding school, he was still wetting his bed at times.

At boarding school, a rough regime and repeated bullying resulted in further withdrawal. Even though he rang home frequently to tell his mother about his unhappiness, she would not really listen. After each holiday he would scream and cry because he did not want to go back, but no one took any notice. He was considered a difficult child who made a great fuss over nothing. However, no one ever bothered to ask him why he so desperately did not want to go back to school.

After 12 sessions of working through his past traumas and releasing pent-up frustration and anger, Paul felt better than he had felt in years. He reported that his energy had started to return, and he began to feel more optimistic about the future again.

ANXIETY

Anxiety is a fear that is not necessarily tied to reality. When you are anxious, you are imagining what might go wrong in the future and you are also mulling over what has gone wrong in the past. This preoccupation with frightening thoughts results in a sometimes permanent state of fright or great agitation.

Some of the main features of anxiety are:

- constant feelings of vague fear

- physical tension

- irritability

- lack of concentration

- problems sleeping

- feeling tired all the time

- irregular breathing pattern
- irregular heart beat
- low stress threshold
- restlessness.

You can see that quite a few of these symptoms overlap with those of depression – as do the reasons why anxiety can develop. The inability to accept and constructively express negative emotions is certainly a strong contributory factor. If you cannot allow anger, you are without a defence mechanism – a bit like a tortoise without its carapace. If you cannot accept your anger it means that anyone can do with you what they will because you are unable to stand up for yourself and stop them. If, however, you can use your anger constructively, you can relax and sleep well at night because you know that if anything needs your attention, if anything goes wrong tomorrow, you will see to it and sort it out, so you do not have to mull over possible disasters all the time.

There is also a personality element in anxiety. Some people are more prone to react anxiously than others, so they are more likely to develop an anxiety problem than others.

Case History: Anxiety

Linda felt constantly irritable and restless, and reported that she worried to such an extent that she had developed severe sleeping problems. She had two young children and had had to cope on her own ever since her husband had left her two years previously for another woman. Her constant anxiety, together with many sleepless nights, had considerably drained her energy. She felt at the end of her tether and finally decided to seek help.

Her earlier childhood background was fairly uneventful; problems only started occurring a year after she had got married. Her husband had been a taciturn person who was given to frequent sarcastic comments on what he called Linda's inadequacies. After four years of marriage she had lost all confidence and had started believing her husband's criticisms. She became more hesitant about making decisions and grew more and more anxious. When he finally left her, she felt it was the last straw – she had to be really useless if she could not even hang on to her husband!

In hypnosis, we worked through her marriage history and gradually Linda recognized that it had in fact been her husband who was inadequate. She began to realize that she had done very well in her marriage, considering she had a difficult husband. With this realization her confidence returned and her anxiety disappeared.

PHOBIAS AND PANIC ATTACKS

A phobia is an excessive, irrational fear which is triggered off by a particular object, activity or situation. Psychologists commonly differentiate between three kinds of phobias – specific phobias, social phobias and agoraphobia (a fear of panic attacks).

A specific phobia is directed towards one particular object such as birds, moths or thunder, for example, although it can also be directed towards a particular situation such as heights. The fear in specific phobias is that of being killed or injured if you get close to the object of your phobia.

With social phobias, on the other hand, the fear centres around embarrassing yourself in the presence of other people. Because of this fear, sufferers are often unable to use public toilets or to eat in restaurants, pubs or other public spaces.

The third type of phobia, agoraphobia, is characterized by a fear of leaving the house, of being alone (even in the house) and of travelling any significant distance from home. Agoraphobic fear is essentially a fear of experiencing a panic attack and not having anyone nearby to help you. This is why panic attack sufferers will avoid public transport, crowds, theatres and cinemas, as well as busy roads. Some sufferers become so anxious about the outside world that they cannot leave their homes any more.

The main features of a phobia are as follows:

- The fear is persistent over a long period of time.

- The fear is unreasonable.

- Knowing that the fear is unreasonable does not help the sufferer stop being afraid.

- Normal daily routines are disrupted because of the phobia.

- Sufferers experience great anxiety or panic if confronted with the feared object, activity or situation.

- In the case of panic attacks there is usually a very strong physical reaction, including trembling, palpitations, feeling rooted to the spot or feeling as if you were going to die. In some cases, a sufferer may even faint.

A panic attack is the explosion of an accumulation of fear which is sometimes mistaken for a heart attack because of all the accompanying physical symptoms.

With a client who has a phobia or a history of panic attacks, the therapist is likely to ask a number of questions, not all of which are directly related to the client's fear. In order to determine which approach is the most useful one – suggestions, desensitization or analysis – the therapist will want to find out whether there has been a lot of stress in the client's life before the onset of the phobia or panic attacks. Stress that has been repressed over a long period of time can surface as a phobia or panic attack at a much later stage, which makes recognizing the source of the phobia or panic attacks very difficult for the sufferer.

Your relationship with your partner might be deteriorating and you may feel that there is a danger that it will break apart, but you may soldier on and never discuss your problems with your partner or anyone else. Even though you consciously suppress the emotional stress the relationship is causing you, subconsciously pressure starts building up, and this is discharged when you cannot handle the volume of pressure any more. If this pressure-discharge happens to take place while you are on the motorway, for example, you are likely to connect this panicky feeling with driving and in future try and avoid fast roads.

Another way in which a phobia can build up is by a series of unpleasant experiences that have resulted in excessive anxiety. You may have had a difficult time at school, being put down by teachers or bullied by classmates. These experiences, especially if they happened repeatedly, can later lead to a great fear of doing anything where you might be the centre of attention, such as eating in public or delivering a presentation in front of a group of people.

Phobias and fears can also be copied from another person. If you have seen your mother lose control at the sight of a spider, you may well 'learn' to be afraid of spiders yourself – because they were obviously something to be terrified of, judging by your mother's reaction ...

Strong fears can also be caused by past trauma which the client may or may not remember. Especially in the case where a memory is no longer consciously available, the therapist will consider using analytical hypnotherapy to uncover what lies at the bottom of the fear so that the traumatic event can be worked through and the emotional ties severed that still bind the client to that event.

Case History: Phobia

Constance had been developing a great fear of lifts and trains over a period of six years. She had managed to avoid these situations successfully for many years, but was no longer able to do so after she changed jobs. Her new office was on the 10th floor of a large office block, plus she was now required to go on frequent business trips by train.

While taking Constance's background history I learned that her fears had started when both she and her husband had lost their jobs within the space of two months. Constance eventually managed to find employment, but her husband remained unemployed. She now found herself in a high-pressure profession with very little support from her husband, so that she had to work long hours only to come home and tend to the children and the household as well.

Constance's main issue in connection with her phobias was that other people would stare at her if she had a panic attack on a train or in a lift. In hypnosis we traced this fear back to the age of eight, when she had been accused of stealing another pupil's pencil case. As the teacher accused her in front of the whole class, all the children looked at Constance. She had felt devastated and very upset. When the pencil case turned up after a few days, nobody bothered to apologize to Constance for having wrongly accused her.

Once this memory had come to light and a few more memories had been worked through, Constance made good progress and soon mastered her phobias. She also became more confident as a consequence of her sessions and managed to persuade her husband to be more helpful at home.

WEIGHT CONTROL
AND EATING DISORDERS

As the old saying goes, food stays in your mouth two seconds, in your stomach two hours and on your hips two years. Extra pounds can creep up on you over a period of weeks and months, and whereas a pound or two may not be a problem, extra pounds can add up after a while. Many people are perfectly capable of sensibly controlling their weight while enjoying their food. Even though many women moan about their weight, most of them have quite a realistic body image.

However, more serious imbalances in eating habits are often a sign that there is a corresponding imbalance on the emotional side.

The main features of an eating disorder are one or several of the following symptoms:

- living to eat rather than eating to live

- obsessional calorie counting

- continuous dieting

- feeling fat no matter how thin you are (anorexia)

- feeling guilty about eating (anorexia, bulimia)

- bingeing and then taking laxatives or making yourself sick (bulimia)

- regularly using food as a source of comfort

- regularly using food to reduce anxiety or anger

- concealing from others what or how much you eat

- hiding food (bulimia)

- exercising excessively (anorexia, bulimia).

Weight control is one of the classic problems that clients see a hypnotherapist with. However, not all weight problems are the same. In straightforward cases the clients have slipped into bad eating habits which they find hard to break. This type of overweight problem is often easily remedied with suggestion therapy and a back-up tape which the clients can use at home.

Overeating can be more than a bad habit, however, and therefore more complex to deal with than, for example, smoking. You can live without smoking, but you cannot live without eating. Eating is a matter of physical and emotional equilibrium; unless there is a certain degree of harmony within a person, eating can easily get out of balance. Stress affects people in various ways – some people cannot eat when they are upset, others, on the contrary, will overeat. If emotional stress gets to be too much a more severe eating disorder, compulsive in nature, can develop.

A real eating disorder is not always easy to spot for someone on the outside, as many compulsive eaters and all bulimics are secretive about their problem. People who suffer from bulimia are rarely overweight. They usually have a history of anorexia before they became bulimic. Once they have reached the bulimia stage, they appear to eat more or less normally, but in reality they are secretly bingeing and then making themselves sick. After their initial relief of having rid themselves of the food they have binged, they then torture themselves with feelings of guilt and shame.

Not so with anorexia. Sufferers are pleased with their non-eating and compulsive exercising; it is very easy for the outside world to detect that something is very wrong because the anorexic person is so painfully thin. As anorexics constantly feel they are too fat they do not want to stop starving themselves, and therefore very rarely come for therapy, whereas bulimics, compulsive eaters and overeaters are among those who are more likely to seek treatment.

Where suggestion therapy is sufficient for clients with habitual rather than compulsive eating problems, any of the more serious eating disorders will require an analytical approach.

The reasons for overweight are in 99 per cent of cases emotional or habitual, and only in 1 per cent of cases physical. With eating disorders, the reason is always emotional.

Here are a few possible reasons that can lead to overeating or an eating disorder:

- coming from a family where several members overeat

- stress brought on by overwork

- stress from emotional overload

- being in an unsatisfactory or abusive relationship

- wanting to punish yourself for being needy (bulimia)

- seeking autonomy (anorexia, bulimia)

- power struggles in the family (anorexia)

- an overtly or covertly domineering mother

- fashion and advertising suggesting that only thin is beautiful

- fear of sex

- fear of growing up

- depression

- anxiety

- feelings of helplessness and vulnerability
- sexual abuse.

Eating too much or too little has symbolic meaning; it is the task of the hypnotherapist to find out what function the overeating or starvation has in the client's life. Any symptom, no matter how bizarre it seems, serves a function, be it comfort, protection or otherwise. It is necessary to enable the client to achieve protection or comfort in a different and more positive way, and in this context past traumas need to be sorted out and confidence built so that the client can let go of the eating crutch.

Case History: Bulimia

Janet was a highly successful executive with a great deal of responsibility. She worked long hours, even on weekends, and had to attend numerous business lunches each week. These official lunches were a problem because Janet was bulimic. She had to eat in public because everyone else did, but at the same time she did not feel she should. So, whenever she could, she would find an opportunity to disappear and make herself sick.

During her teens Janet had suffered from anorexia and had lived exclusively on fruit, starving herself down to only 6 stone (38 kg).

Like many bulimics, Janet had a very strong need to control and an inability to relax. She was highly efficient in a driven, uncompromising and self-effacing way. Everyone and everything else was more important and took priority over her own feelings, and she worked so much that there was really no time to think about herself.

As we found out in analytical hypnotherapy sessions, Janet felt very isolated as a child. Her father, whom she felt close to, had worked away a lot, and her mother had been a difficult

60 woman, driven by her tempers and always suspecting her husband of having affairs. Janet's two brothers diverted themselves from the difficulties at home by playing with other boys in the neighbourhood, but there were no girls so Janet was stuck at home with her mother, who was so completely wrapped up in her own problems that she quite forgot about her daughter. Janet withdrew into herself and read day and night to overcome her loneliness.

Her parents expected her to look after her brothers while they went away on reconciliation weekends to try and patch up their marriage, leaving 13-year-old Janet in charge of the boys. Janet felt burdened by the great responsibility of it all but did not feel she could tell her mother about her difficulties with the boys when they were naughty because she did not want to tell on them.

Then a rumour started that Janet's father had molested a girl from Janet's school. As a consequence, Janet now also became an outsider at school, where the others shunned her for what her father was supposed to have done. Shortly after this incident, Janet stopped eating and became anorexic.

In her sessions we worked through her feelings about her parents and her overriding sense of loneliness and isolation. After three sessions Janet already noted a decrease in the number of times she felt compelled to make herself sick; after 15 sessions she could eat normally.

CONFIDENCE AND SELF-WORTH

There is one fundamental difference between a lack of confidence and lack of self-worth – when you lack confidence, you feel unable to do one or several things in life, whereas when you lack self-worth, you feel you *do not deserve* to do one or several things in life. A lack of self-worth will therefore automatically include a lack of confidence, whereas someone can lack confidence without being low in self-esteem.

The main features of a lack in confidence are:

- remaining passive in certain situations where being active would improve life for you

- not saying what you think where it would be appropriate to do so

- not standing by what you said earlier

- always putting others first

- an inability to say no

- an inability to make decisions

- doing as you are told but resenting it

- shouting or getting angry when you want something.

The main features of a lack of self-worth are:

- all the above points, and

- feeling that anything bad that happens to you is your fault

- feeling that anything bad that happens to you is a punishment for being such a worthless person

- putting yourself down in your thoughts

- putting yourself down in front of others

- self-abuse (smoking, drinking, drugs)

- choosing abusive partners and staying with them because you feel they are what you deserve

- rejecting people who are nice to you because you assume they are either lying to you or are too stupid to see how worthless you are

- in extreme cases, self-mutilation or suicide.

A lack of confidence in a mild form is something that most people will have experienced at one time or another, typically during the teenage years when you have to learn how to deal with all the physical changes going on in your body while at the same time trying to join the adult world. But even later on, when we have become proficient in many areas of life, we can still be unconfident about particular aspects of ourselves. Maybe we cannot cope with public speaking; maybe we feel intimidated by people in authority; or maybe we find it difficult to complain when we are dissatisfied with a service.

If your lack of confidence is restricted to only one such area, a hypnotherapist will in all likelihood give you some suggestion therapy and possibly also a tape to reinforce the suggestions at home. Only if there are a cluster of confidence problems will the therapist start looking more closely at the underlying reasons by using analysis.

Among the reasons for low confidence can be one or several of the following:

- lack of attention and encouragement from your parents in childhood

- one or several negative experiences when you have tried to be assertive

- parents who were unconfident themselves

- living in an environment where dissenting opinions are not tolerated or are ridiculed

- guilt about something that has happened in the past

- criticism or disapproval in childhood, adolescence and/or with your present partner

- parents who argued a lot

- parents who divorced, and having a divorced parent who did not stay in touch with you once he or she had left home.

With low self-esteem, a hypnotherapist would be more likely to go for an analytical approach straight away to find out what had happened in the client's life that brought about such a negative self-image. Although it is true to say that your personality type plays a part in how you deal with life situations, there is always also an external component that will influence your view of yourself. You may have been shy since birth, but that in itself is no barrier to growing up into a person who likes him- or herself. It is the way others react to you that will determine whether you develop self-worth or not.

Here are a few reasons that can (but do not have to) lie at the bottom of a lack of self-worth:

- being humiliated frequently

- having suffered verbal, physical or sexual abuse

- having been emotionally neglected over long periods as a child

- growing up in a home where no close one-to-one relationship with an adult could be built up

- seeing someone else in the family being subjected to verbal, physical or sexual abuse and feeling unable to help

- having parents who fought physically

- never getting help from anyone, no matter how upset you were about a problem.

Self-worth begins to develop very early on in life and, until it has become firmly established, it is very vulnerable to outside events. Children relate everything around them to themselves. As children are dependent on their parents for food, shelter, love and recognition, any events that jeopardize their emotional safety will be upsetting to them. As children begin to realize that there are lots of things they are unable to do and get wrong, they automatically assume that anything that goes wrong in their environment is their fault: Maybe my parents would not fight all the time if I were not around? Maybe my father would not be in such a bad mood if I were prettier/quicker/cleverer? An adult outsider can see that the parents fight because they are incompatible or that the father criticizes because he has an inferiority complex himself; a child can only blame him- or herself.

Case History: Self-worth

Peter was 25 when he came for treatment. He had been in prison several times for various serious thefts he had committed. Apart from a fundamental sense of self-loathing, he also suffered from anxiety and depression.

As we started exploring his lack of self-worth, we came across a long string of unhappy memories. Growing up in the countryside, Peter was brought up by his mother and grandmother, his father making only occasional appearances, usually when drunk. Peter's mother and grandmother did not see eye to eye and vented their frustrations on Peter by verbally attacking him. In addition, Peter was beaten up regularly by his elder brother and on many occasions by his father. As the youngest of the family, it seemed to Peter that the dissatisfaction of the entire world descended on him on a daily basis. It was as if he were the family punch bag that got knocked around whenever anyone was angry or dissatisfied. He could not remember a single happy event in his early life.

Peter started occasionally stealing small amounts of money from his mother and grandmother, until one day he was caught. He consequently got a beating from his grandmother, his brother and his father, and his grandmother announced publicly that her grandson was a thief and would always be a thief. Peter was devastated and overwhelmed by guilt. Whatever self-esteem had survived the beatings quickly disappeared after this public character assassination. Peter had nothing more to lose, so he followed the path that had been predicted for him – he became a thief on a grand scale and started to burgle houses.

Our hypno-analytical sessions became an agonizing search for the good in him. In the process it was necessary to have a closer look at his parents, grandmother and brother. It took quite a few sessions until Peter could allow himself to contemplate the possibility that others might have been out of order in the way they treated him, so used was he to blaming himself for anything that happened to him. But finally the breakthrough was achieved. Peter started building up self-esteem and decided to enrol for a college course, which he completed after three years.

SEXUAL PROBLEMS

Enjoyment and full achievement of sexual pleasure is a natural process which needs to be allowed to function spontaneously. The normal sexual response cycle consists of the initial arousal stage, followed by a plateau where the arousal has reached a peak and remains stable for a little while, which is then released into an orgasm. The orgasm is a pleasurable feeling which in a woman involves involuntary contractions of the muscles surrounding the vagina, and in a man the involuntary contractions of the penis and ejaculation of semen. The orgasm is followed by a phase termed resolution where both men and women lose their responsiveness to sexual stimulation for a while.

When this natural cycle is disrupted or does not take place at all, one of the following symptoms can indicate that there is a problem:

- little or no desire for sex

- total rejection of sex as disgusting

- inability to achieve orgasm

- inability to sustain erection long enough to penetrate

- ejaculation before or shortly after penetration

- great muscle tension in the vagina so that penetration becomes very painful or impossible.

There can be a number of causes for sexual problems, and not all of them are psychological. When a man's penile arteries are blocked, this will inhibit or even prevent an erection. Similarly, a low level of hormones can cause a lack of sexual interest in both men and women, as can the intake of medication to treat high blood-pressure, and other drugs.

However, in the majority of cases there is a strong psycho-logical component. Because the sexual response cycle happens naturally once appropriate stimulation is administered, it is vulnerable to interruption through stress or worry. In order to achieve a complete cycle you need to be able to get absorbed in the sexual act; otherwise, the interference of other thoughts will disrupt the process. This means that sexual problems can begin to appear at those times when you are experiencing upset in your life. This can be a sudden change in your circumstances, such as a new job or a new baby, or it can happen because you have just been made redundant or are experiencing great financial difficulties.

Another reason for sexual problems can be the fact that there are difficulties within the relationship. Even though some partners thrive on arguments because they tend to make them up in bed, others find that arguing turns them off sex altogether.

Also, if a woman has a partner who is very inexperienced, sex can be less than satisfactory for her. This obviously has nothing to do with stress or an emotional problem on the woman's part.

All the aforementioned causes for sexual problems are triggered by external circumstances. This means that the problem is likely to resolve itself once you have learned to cope better with stress and relax more, or when you have sorted out your relationship problems. In these cases, counselling or relaxation exercises can often resolve the problem quite easily.

Matters become more complex when the cause lies inside the person who experiences the sexual difficulties. This is often due to a strict upbringing with strong moral overtones. Families or schools that are very religious can often imply, directly or indirectly, that sex is bad or dirty. Masturbation, which for children is a necessary part of developing sexual maturity, is still often regarded as wrong, and if youngsters are subjected to guilty feelings over their growing interest in their own body and in sexual matters generally, this can lead to difficulties later on. In extreme cases, sex is so much linked with guilt that sexual gratification can only be experienced when it is administered as punishment (masochism).

Witnessing one's parents making love can also be strongly disruptive to normal sexual functioning as an adult. A child who is too young to understand what is going on will find this a very frightening experience: the noises, movements and positions can make it seem as though one parent is doing something terrible to the other. It all looks out of control and frightening; to a sensitive child this can be a traumatic experience.

However, the most grave trauma to a child is that of being sexually molested or abused. As already discussed in the section on confidence and self-worth (*page 60*), children always blame themselves for what is happening to them. The experience of sexual abuse does not just leave the child ashamed and guilty, but also with a contorted view of sexuality and sexual intercourse.

In all cases where the sexual problem originates from within the person, the feelings of guilt need to be resolved before the client can experience an improvement.

Case History: Premature Ejaculation

Michael was in his mid-thirties when he came for treatment. He was divorced from his wife, had lived on his own for three years and had recently started a new relationship. He was very happy with his new girlfriend, whom he described as 'gorgeous', but unfortunately he felt he could not perform in bed. He got overexcited and ejaculated far too early. Luckily, his girlfriend was very understanding, but he was worried that she might lose respect for him unless this matter changed for the better soon. But the harder he tried to restrain his ejaculation, the less he could do so. The problem had been going on for eight weeks when he first came to see me.

I explained to him that this was definitely only a temporary problem, which would go away as soon as he stopped trying to make it go away. As he had been able to perform well with his wife and with girlfriends before her, he just needed to get back into the swing of what he was capable of doing anyway.

I spent the first session teaching Michael self-hypnosis for relaxation, which he took to quite easily. I also gave him a self-hypnosis relaxation tape as homework, to be listened to every day. When he came for his second session he reported that there had already been some improvement.

During the second session I helped Michael into hypnosis and encouraged him to remember the most exciting and satisfying sex he had ever had. He was not required to say anything, but just to immerse himself in the memory. Soon, a wide smile appeared on his face and he breathed a deep sigh of relief. He blushed a little as he came out of hypnosis, and left hurriedly.

Three days later he rang up, elated, to say everything was fine and he that would not need any further sessions.

OBSESSIONS AND COMPULSIONS

People suffering from an obsession have a persistent idea or thought in their minds which frightens them. This could be, for example, 'I'm going to have an accident today' or 'The house is full of germs' or 'I am going to hurt someone.' Even though sufferers can see that this thought is irrational, they still cannot stop themselves from thinking it. As this thought or idea causes great anxiety, obsessive people often try to counteract it by going through a compulsive action which they have to perform like a ritual every time the obsessive thought comes into their minds. The compulsive action reassures sufferers for a little while, until the thought reappears and the compulsive action has to be repeated.

Some people have a milder form of obsessive compulsive

disorder which is termed 'obsessive compulsive tendencies'. These people might find that when they are stressed they check and re-check locks or taps, but as soon as the stress has passed they can stop their compulsive behaviour. However, people who have the more severe version are at such a high level of tension that they find it impossible to abandon their ritualistic thoughts and actions, even when life is running smoothly.

An obsessive compulsive disorder can show itself in a great number of ways. The following list (which is not comprehensive) gives you a few symptoms and examples:

- not treading on the cracks in the pavement (mild form)

- avoiding certain colours or numbers at all cost

- checking and re-checking that you have locked the doors/turned off the cooker/closed all the windows/turned off all water taps, etc.

- having to have things in a particular order in the house

- constantly cleaning the house

- constantly washing your hands

- counting and re-counting money in your purse

- exaggerated concern with dirt and germs

- exaggerated concern with body wastes

- having to touch certain items (for example the doorknob) a certain number of times before you enter or leave a room

- having to say a particular phrase in your mind to counteract the frightening thought

- fear of harming yourself or others

- fear of blurting out obscenities

- inability to control obsessive thoughts or compulsive actions

- having obsessive thoughts/compulsive actions that take over your life and dictate your daily routines.

People with obsessive compulsive disorders are often (but not always) of a particular personality type. They may find it difficult to express warm emotions, they put work before pleasure and are generally very critical of themselves and others, with a perfectionist streak and a tendency to be overconscientious and inflexible. Their inflexibility in particular can make it somewhat difficult to treat these clients. However, both hypnoanalysis and behaviour therapy have been shown to achieve very good results, and follow-ups suggest that these positive outcomes are lasting.

An obsessive compulsive disorder can come seemingly out of the blue, without an obvious reason. All you notice is that you suddenly have a very frightening thought in your mind which you need to get rid of because it upsets you so much, so you do something 'magical' such as saying a certain word or phrase to yourself or doing a particular thing, such as going through a doorway backwards a certain number of times to prevent the terrible thought from coming true.

Similar to panic attacks, obsessive compulsive disorders are usually preceded by one or several stressful life events which have already heightened the client's fear level. Sometimes, this life event can be an illness, a crisis situation at home or stress at work. People most susceptible to the disorder are those who have low confidence and/or low self-esteem and are therefore generally of an anxious disposition.

In order to help a client overcome an obsessive and/or

compulsive problem, a therapist will aim at sorting out the fundamental anxieties that caused the stress overload before the onset of the disorder. By working through past trauma, confidence and self-esteem can be established and the client gains a stronger feeling of control. As a consequence, the obsessive thoughts begin to disappear, and with them the compulsive actions.

Case History: Obsessive Thoughts

Maureen had been married for six years and had two little daughters. Two years previously she had started suffering from the disturbing thoughts that she would harm her children. On the one hand, she knew that she would never ever do that, but that knowledge did not help make the obsessional thoughts go away. She was very distraught about the thoughts and spent a lot of time assuring me that they were only thoughts and that she could never do any harm to her children. Maureen was deeply ashamed about her problem and was afraid that she was going mad. She had coped so far by trying to keep herself very busy, but whenever there was a lull in activity the thoughts came back.

On taking Maureen's background history we found that two things had happened shortly before the onset of her obsessive thoughts. Six months before the problems started she had found out that her husband was having an affair. She was upset and became very insecure, searching for a reason why her husband might do this, and at the same time feeling betrayed by him. But since the children adored their father, she felt she needed to swallow her anger. After the initial confession, the affair was never mentioned again but, for Maureen, the matter remained very much on her mind. She spent a lot of time 'explaining away' her husband's behaviour by finding fault with herself.

A few weeks after that a neighbour had told Maureen that a six-year-old boy they both knew had been murdered, apparently by his mother. Even though this was never proved, the image stuck in Maureen's mind – a mother murdering her child. Maureen now started experiencing the frightening thoughts of herself with a knife in her hand, harming her own children. No matter how many examples she had of how caring she was in reality, she lived in fear that one day these thoughts would turn into reality.

As we were going through Maureen's memories in hypnosis, we came across a great number of earlier occasions on which Maureen had been treated like the Cinderella of her family when she was small. She was rarely praised and often blamed, whereas her older sister could do no wrong. She had become unconfident and withdrawn by the time she married, but gradually found her feet as a wife and mother, until her husband's affair shattered her fragile confidence.

We worked through several of her childhood traumas as well as the unfinished business of her husband's infidelity. As she was describing her feelings towards him when she found out about the affair, she said she could have 'stuck a knife into him'. So here was the knife of her obsessional thoughts! It appeared that she was unable to vent her anger (= knife) towards her husband for fear that he might leave her, so the feeling was subconsciously diverted towards her children instead, the link being provided by the shocking real-life story about the murdered little boy.

Once Maureen had vented her anger in hypnosis towards the people who had inspired it, she reported a marked decrease in her obsessional thinking. She became more confident and was happy to see the negative thoughts peter out.

PAIN CONTROL

Hypnotherapy has proved very useful as an anaesthetic in a variety of situations. Here are a few of the most common pain areas that respond to hypnosis:

- burns

- cancer

- phantom pain in an amputated limb

- childbirth

- dental surgery

- general surgery, including Caesarean

- chronic pain brought on by illness.

Some people are allergic to anaesthetics, so hypnosis can function as a substitute. Hypnosis can also replace painkillers and muscle relaxants. It is now a well-established fact that general anaesthesia constitutes a risk as it is a major burden for the body, and chemicals administered before and during an operation remain in the body for years. Hypnosis used as painkiller, anaesthetic or muscle relaxant has none of these undesirable side-effects.

If we were to define the feeling of pain, we would probably call it an unpleasant physical sensation that causes us emotional distress. But what actually happens in the body?

When your skin comes into contact with an injurious object, such as someone else's foot on your toes or the hot oven door against your fingers, microscopic structures in the skin called free nerve endings conduct impulses to the spinal cord via nerve fibres. From the spinal cord, the pain message is relayed to the thalamus in the brain – it is at this moment that you quickly pull your hand away from the oven or tell the other person to get off your foot!

All this takes place within a fraction of a second. In this context, pain is a necessity because it makes sure we get away from the harmful object so that greater injury is prevented.

But pain can also occur as a consequence of damage to the nervous system, either through injury or disease. In these cases, pain can be persistent without serving a purpose. The same situation occurs when someone loses a limb – the person experiences the impression that the limb is still there, and some amputees can even suffer from very unpleasant phantom pain in that lost limb. Again, the pain does not serve any purpose.

However, your pain perception is not only dependent on the sharpness of the impact with a noxious object. There are several other factors that will determine how severely you experience pain. You will remember that in the section about phobias (*page 52*) we established that you can 'catch' a phobic reaction from someone else. The same is true of reactions to pain. If you were brought up among people who made a big fuss when you or they sustained a minor injury, you are more likely to be afraid of pain, and this in turn will make you experience any pain as quite severe.

Your overall state of mind and emotions also play their part. If you feel that you have very little control over your life, if you are dependent on others and if you have low self-esteem, you are much more likely to fear pain and experience it as traumatic than someone who feels confident and in control.

In order to help a client reduce or switch off pain, a hypnotherapist will first of all have to send the client to a GP to check that there are no physical causes for the pain, such as a growth or an illness that has not been diagnosed. Once these possibilities have been ruled out, the hypnotherapist is likely to induce a comfortable state of hypnosis and then proceed to work with imagery.

When the client is being prepared for an operation, the therapist might ask which scenario the client finds the most relaxing. Some people are happiest in the mountains, others by a lake or on the beach. This preferred scenery is then introduced after the initial hypnotic induction and the client is taught how to immerse him- or herself into that scenery for an extended time.

Case History: Dental Surgery

Stephen was allergic to anaesthetics but had to have some dental surgery done. His dentist, who had trained in hypnotherapy, helped Stephen into hypnosis using the imagery of sailing on a big lake, as this was Stephen's favourite pastime. Over the next two hours Stephen was busy 'sailing', integrating the dentist's lamp into his dream as radiant sunshine and the gurgling sounds of the suction apparatus as the ripples of water against the side of his boat, while the dentist's scalpel was cutting deep into his gums . . .

Where a client suffers from pain caused by illness or injury, including phantom pain in an amputated limb, the hypnotherapist may also suggest that the client imagine the pain as an object. If the pain is experienced as searing, the client might describe it as a ball of flames; if it is a stabbing pain it might be likened to a battery of knives hacking into a particular part of the body, and so on. The client can then learn, in hypnosis, to counteract this image by imposing a soothing image over the painful one. The ball of fire can be gently inserted into a cool mountain of snow; the site of the body suffering blows from the knives can be reinforced so that the knives can do no damage.

Case History: Phantom Pain

Cedric suffered from frequent pain in his amputated hand which even strong painkillers could not control. His doctor referred him to a hypnotherapist who taught Cedric self-hypnosis to relax and bring the pain level down. In hypnosis, the therapist suggested to Cedric that he could feel the pleasurable sensation of stroking a cat's silky fur whenever he thought of his amputated hand. This link between the amputated limb and a pleasant tactile sensation was then anchored with a post-hypnotic suggestion so that Cedric was able to switch off the pain himself as soon as it arose.

It is still not clear how hypnosis can have this effect. Originally it was thought that hypnosis caused the release of the body's own opiates. However, even when hypnotized subjects are given Naloxon, a substance which renders opiates ineffective, they remain resistant to pain. It would appear that focusing on images in hypnosis absorbs a person's concentration to such an extent that the perception of pain is switched off.

PSYCHOSOMATIC DISORDERS

The word *psychosomatic* is applied to conditions where psychological stresses affect the body adversely. We have already looked at the connection between body and mind and how the conscious and subconscious minds interact (*see pages 6–9*). When emotional stress occurs frequently, and particularly if these stressful emotions are not expressed, the autonomic nervous system is on constant alert; this raises blood-pressure and causes the body's glands to secrete more hormones than you need, with the result that the inner organs are under unnecessary strain. For example, if you are angry, your blood-pressure will rise and your heart rate and breathing rate will increase.

Once your anger has abated, these physiological processes reverse themselves. However, if you are chronically angry (and particularly when you are unable to vent that anger), the physical symptoms associated with the angry state persist. With time you become aware of the uncomfortable feelings associated with high blood-pressure, without necessarily being aware of the emotions that have evoked those symptoms in the first place.

Among illnesses and disorders which involve a psychosomatic component are the following:

- high blood-pressure

- asthma

- eczema

- psoriasis

- irritable bowel syndrome (IBS)

- tension headaches

- back and neck pain

- impotence

- dermatitis

- ulcers

- cancer

- multiple sclerosis (MS)

- myalgic encephalomyelitis (ME) and chronic fatigue syndrome (CFS).

With psychosomatic conditions, a hypnotherapist will concentrate on the emotion or emotions that are putting pressure on the body and preventing it from functioning properly. In this context, it is less important where in the body the emotional overload presents itself; what is significant is that the body is reacting to something that is not working on the emotional level. The afflicted organ, be it skin, heart or bowel, just functions as the weakest point, very much like a fuse in a fuse box which blows when there is an electric overload. However, some therapists attach great importance to the kind of psychosomatic illness a patient has, and link certain illnesses to certain emotions. If a client comes with back and neck aches, they might try and find out who in the client's life is a 'pain in the neck'; if a person has an ulcer, the therapist might attribute that to something 'eating' the client; or if a client comes with asthma, they might ask what it is the client needs to get off his or her chest. Often these associations between illness and emotions are quite accurate.

The reasons for psychosomatic disorders can be varied, but they are usually linked to an ongoing stressful life situation which, for one reason or another, sufferers cannot (or feel they should not) air. This can be an untenable situation at work where they are required to do jobs which they have not been trained to do, an unpleasant work atmosphere, frequent arguments at work or at home, feeling burdened by great responsibilities without getting recognition, or aggravation over an ongoing situation such as a long-term project at work or problems with difficult children or difficult parents.

It is really surprising how resilient the body is to stress. Emotional upset often needs to go on for a long time before the body's defenses break down or, to put it more precisely, before we *notice* that our body is suffering from the emotional onslaught. The body has an incredibly efficient way of recuperating, so when we find we cannot recover from an illness this indicates that we must have run down our resources. This is a warning signal that must be taken seriously or we risk even graver physical problems.

Case History: Asthma

Victoria had developed asthma two years previously, about six months after her father had died. She was 38 years of age and working as a counsellor. During the initial consultation Victoria said that she would like to settle down and have a family of her own. Before we started with hypnosis we checked through all the events that had occurred before her breathing problems started. Victoria reported that she had helped to lay a carpet and that the glue used had affected her breathing, but on reflection she decided that that had happened after the asthma had already started, so the fumes from the glue might have made the asthma worse but could not have caused it.

The obvious traumatic event before the asthma was her father's death, but Victoria was not aware that this had been a problem for her. We agreed to double-check this in hypnosis. Victoria went back to the time before her father died and brought up memories of a cantankerous man who kept everyone on their toes with his moods and demands. In order to keep the peace, Victoria had acted as mediator between her father and the rest of the family ever since she had been little. When he finally died, she was upset, but not unduly so as she had never been very close to her father.

However, after her father's death Victoria's mother seemed to require a lot of attention. Victoria found herself travelling up to her mother's every weekend after having done so for the previous two years to help attend to her bedridden father. Working during the week and keeping her mother company on weekends, Victoria still had no opportunity to develop a private life, and she felt that time was running out if she wanted to start her own family. When I pointed out to her that she was looking after everyone else and asked who was looking after her, she burst into tears. Having felt responsible for others' well-being all her life, she felt unable to see to her own happiness.

After the first session Victoria said she could already feel a great weight lifting. She said it was virtually as if she had got something off her chest, and her asthma started improving.

After a few more sessions of strengthening her confidence and letting go of her feelings of guilt for wanting to focus on herself and her own needs, Victoria was able to speak to her mother and explain that she wanted to visit less frequently so she could have a chance of building up a private life.

The asthma continued to improve to such an extent that Victoria did not have to use her inhaler any more.

ENHANCING PERFORMANCE

There are an increasing number of sportsmen and -women today who make use of hypnosis and self-hypnosis to ensure that they are in top form when they have to compete. It is no longer unusual to hear of sports psychologists and hypnotherapists supporting football teams, tennis players, gymnasts, boxers, golfers and runners. It is now understood that it is not enough only to train your body; unless your mind is focused on supporting and reinforcing your body's performance, you will not be able to access your maximum potential. Self-hypnosis through visualization is a popular and effective method used by an increasing number of athletes to refine their technique and to train their minds to see the successful outcome of, say, their golf swing, their gymnastic routine or their game of tennis.

Hypnosis is used to help with the following areas:

- to increase the speed with which you learn new techniques and new skills in your sport

- to improve concentration

- to improve precision

- to heighten awareness of body position during certain movements

- to eliminate fear of failure.

Various experiments have proved that hypnosis can help increase the body's strength and performance, in respect of both sheer physical output and mental attitude. In one experiment subjects were tested for the muscle strength in their dominant arm, depending on whether they were right- or lefthanded. It was found that, on average, lifting strength lay at around 90 pounds. When these subjects were later given suggestions that they were tired and weak, their muscle power decreased to an average of 25 pounds. They were then given the opposite suggestion, namely that they felt in top form and were experiencing an unusual surge of energy in their body; as a result the average of muscle power in the test group rose to an amazing 140 pounds. All this happened within one hour.

The importance of attitude and beliefs was also demonstrated in experiments with runners. A runner who would regularly lose races to a team-mate was given placebo pills (pills without any active ingredients) and told that these pills would help him increase his performance to such an extent that he would be able to overtake his team-mate. Within a short period of time, the runner beat his team-mate in every race they ran. Even when he stopped taking the 'pills', he maintained his higher performance levels.

There have been concerns that the use of hypnosis could lead to over-exertion of the body and therefore to serious damage and burn-out, but these fears have proved unfounded. What appears to happen is that hypnotic suggestions enhance performance by removing the mental barriers that prevent the display of full muscle power, coordination and concentration, rather than adding anything artificial by giving the athlete something extra that was not there in the first place. In other words, hypnosis helps bring out the best in an athlete.

It goes without saying that you need to train regularly and have a certain amount of talent for your chosen area of sport, but provided these basic ingredients are there, hypnosis can considerably improve your performance and open up the way to the very top of your field.

Other areas where hypnosis can help enhance performance are:

- improving memory

- improving creativity

- overcoming stage fright in actors, singers, dancers and other performers

- improving test/exam results through heightened concentration and elimination of 'nerves'

- removing writer's block

- improving attention span

- accelerating learning.

Case History: Golf
Bill had been playing golf ever since he had retired three years previously, and had been making good progress until he 'lost it' during his first club tournament. He had become very nervous

when he felt all eyes on him, and ever since then his game had deteriorated because he expected to do badly. Now, he hardly ever accomplished an acceptable swing, and this of course greatly diminished his enjoyment of golf.

In his three hypnotherapy sessions Bill learned to relax properly and then to create a mental 'tunnel vision' which helped him to concentrate totally on his swing. He used as his foundation the memory of what he had been able to achieve in the past when it came to handling the club skilfully. He then took himself through all the details of executing a perfect swing: the correct position, the feel of balance, the position of his hands on the club, the movement of his upper body, hips and arms, and the precise motion when he hit the ball.

Bill practised his golf swing in his mind, using self-hypnosis, and soon reported that he was back to his old form again on the green.

WHAT TO EXPECT WHEN
YOU GO FOR TREATMENT

As with any form of treatment that deals with human emotions, it is of utmost importance that you see a competent practitioner if you decide to try hypnotherapy to help with your problems. But how do you know that a therapist is competent? The Yellow Pages are full of advertisements for hypnotherapists, and some of them look impressive because of their size and elaborate layout, just as some hypnotherapists seem to be very well qualified judging by the string of letters after their names. Unfortunately, neither expensive advertising nor the letters after someone's name will guarantee that the practitioner you see will be competent. Even a good school of hypnotherapy will produce some bad hypnotherapists, just as a mediocre school can bring forth some good, competent therapists who realize the limitations of their schooling and go on to other courses to further their knowledge. For it is not just a matter of learning about the various methods of inducing hypnosis, applying suggestions and working through memories, it is also necessary to have sorted out your own problems before you start treating other people. Not all schools require their students to undergo a training analysis, but this should always be part of becoming a therapist. In addition to the training analysis, new therapists should also be supervised, at least during their first year of practice, to make sure they get regular feedback and back-up from an experienced senior therapist. Many newly qualified therapists give up their practice because they cannot stand the enormous responsibilities that the job carries with it.

Finally, a therapist needs to be able to relate positively to clients, and that is a personal quality which not everyone has. Being a good hypnotherapist, or good at any other form of psychotherapy for that matter, requires having a genuine interest in others, being able to think on your feet, being confident and in control of your own life, and having the ability to leave clients' problems at the office and not take them home with you. As you can see, this is quite a formidable list of necessary qualifications and qualities.

The best way of choosing a hypnotherapist is obviously through recommendation; however, this is not always possible. In order to help you in your choice of practitioner this chapter details what you can expect, from the initial consultation to the actual treatment itself. On *pages 113 – 16* there is also a list of questions you should ask yourself or the therapist before you commit to a course of treatment.

BEFORE YOU MAKE AN APPOINTMENT

Most people will look for a hypnotherapist in the area where they live or work, unless the therapist has been recommended, in which case they may feel it is worth travelling further out.

If none of your friends or family can recommend a therapist, ask your GP. These days, general practitioners often have leaflets available describing the hypnotherapy options available locally. If your doctor does, always ask whether other patients have seen the hypnotherapist and what the results were. That way you avoid going to someone who has just left leaflets in the waiting room without asking permission, or to someone who is not actually known to the GP.

Another source of information can be your local paper or your local business directory. Pick out two or three names of therapists near you. In doing this, take into consideration whether you would be more comfortable with a male or a female therapist. Ring up and take note of how the phone is answered: by an actual person, by an answering machine, or not at all.

If the phone is answered personally, you have either been lucky to get the hypnotherapist directly, or the therapist has a receptionist and is working in a clinic with other practitioners. If you get an answering machine, do not hang up! Instead, take this opportunity to listen carefully to the message. Does it sound professional? Do you like the voice? The majority of hypnotherapists work on their own, without a receptionist to take their calls, and so have to rely on an answering machine while they are with a client.

If there is neither an answering machine nor a direct answer to your phone call, and instead the phone just keeps ringing, the therapist is possibly not very professional. Try again the next day; if you still cannot get through, pick another name from the phone book.

Some therapists will offer to send you a brochure; others do not produce any written information about themselves. It can be useful to see a brochure first because it can give you more information about practitioners, their qualifications and how they work. The quality of the brochure can also give you an initial impression of a therapist's professionalism. However, the ultimate test comes when you actually meet the therapist personally, so all these preliminary indications should be noted but not made into the ultimate determining factors when it comes to choosing a therapist.

If you leave your name and phone number on the answering machine, you should get a call back the same day during office hours or the next day at the latest. Please do not expect the hypnotherapist to ring you late in the evening at home or on a weekend; not every therapist works on Saturdays. Provided you ring on a weekday, you can expect a return call within 24 hours.

Unless you are sure that you want straightforward suggestion therapy (to help you to quit smoking, for example), *always* make an appointment for an initial consultation first, especially if you have not seen a brochure. If you feel anxious or unconfident about going on your own, take a friend with you to the initial meeting so that the two of you can confer afterwards. As a matter of courtesy you should ask the hypnotherapist whether it is all right to bring someone else along. In this context, please be aware that most therapists will not agree to having another person in the room once the actual sessions start – unless the client is a child, in which case a parent or guardian must always be present during treatment. The reason for not allowing another person to be present while an adult client is receiving treatment is that it hampers progress. The client is going to be much more reluctant to be open about memories, especially embarrassing or painful ones, if someone other than the therapist is present.

THE INITIAL CONSULTATION

Some hypnotherapists work from home, others from business premises. Even though a practice away from home may initially seem more professional, do not be put off if you find that the address turns out to be the therapist's home. Some houses are spacious enough to use one room as the practice, and that is fine. What is more important is that the place is reasonably quiet. Screaming children in the next room and a friendly dog who comes walking in and out of the room during the consultation are not what you want if you are expected to pay for your sessions.

The initial consultation is the time to ask all the questions you want, and it is also when the therapist can decide whether it is possible to take you on. At this first meeting the therapist will want to make sure that your problem is one that can be treated with hypnotherapy, and will also want to explain a bit more about how he or she works. For you, this is an opportunity to ask how long the therapist has been in practice and, if it has been for less than a year, whether he or she is working under supervision. You will also be able to see how many diplomas are on the walls. Generally, it is a good sign if a practitioner has passed through several courses because it shows that the therapist keeps working on his or her skills. You should also find out whether the therapist has professional indemnity insurance. This insurance will cover the therapist if any claims are brought against him or her. It is also a sign that the therapist belongs to a recognized body of hypnotherapists, as insurance companies will not insure individuals working 'freelance', as it were.

The initial consultation will normally not involve hypnosis; its function is for you and the therapist to get the information you both need. Keep the description of your problem short; there will be time to go into more detail once you have started the first session. Remember that this is your opportunity to evaluate whether you feel comfortable with the therapist, whether you feel he or she is trustworthy, comes across as professional and seems to know what he or she is talking about.

This is also the time to discuss fees. Many therapists offer a sliding scale for treatment that takes longer than three sessions; often their brochure will have told you this already. Some therapists charge a 'case fee' which is payable before or after the first session and is usually a larger sum of money than that for a regular session. If this is what your potential therapist does, ask what you will get for your money. If this money is just for the therapist taking you on, you might want to reconsider. However, if the money pays for an extra-long first session and also covers for the therapist's time to work through your background history, a case fee can be justified and acceptable.

It is not advisable to part with a lump sum for the whole course of treatment up front. For one thing, there is no way anyone can predict exactly how many sessions you will need, and also you may be dissatisfied with the therapist's conduct after a few sessions but unwilling to leave because you have made this financial commitment. The usual method is to pay session by session as you go along, or to pay one session in advance. This latter method is a safeguard for the therapist, to ensure that you give at least 24 hours' notice if you cannot attend a session; if you do not give enough notice or just do not turn up, you forfeit the advanced payment.

At the time of writing, hypnotherapy sessions can cost anything between £15 and £60 per session, with case fees lying between £80 and £150.

BACKGROUND HISTORY

If your problem requires more lengthy treatment, the hypnotherapist is likely to want to know more about your childhood and adolescence and also about your present circumstances, for example whether you are in a relationship and, if so, whether you are happy in it.

Do not be put out if you are also asked some personal questions such as whether you have ever had an abortion or miscarriage. This is not meant to be intrusive; the therapist needs to know about such events, as they can cause serious trauma which can linger in the mind and cause feelings of guilt, inadequacy, grief and emotional problems later on.

Some therapists will only take a brief background history, others go into great detail. Another school of thought believes that it is not necessary to know anything at all about clients' lives and circumstances. None of these opinions is strictly right or wrong; they are simply different ways of operating.

However, taking a background history has various advantages. It allows the therapist to gain some insight into your past and some understanding of how you might have developed your self-image and beliefs. By finding out more about your childhood and adolescence, as well as your present circumstances, the experienced therapist will already have an idea of which areas of your life need to be focused on during therapy. If, for example, a client clearly lacks self-confidence and mentions that he was bullied at school, the therapist can check out these school memories in hypnosis to see whether the bullying was indeed instrumental in affecting the client's confidence. Also, any positive memories about achievements in the past can be used during therapy to help the client build a better self-image or to help him master a current problem. Remember the first case history about smoking earlier in this book (*see page 45*)? This was an instance where a past achievement was successfully used as the foundation for a present solution to the client's problem.

When giving your background history it makes sense to be as honest as possible. Often we feel awkward about certain times and events in our lives, but as you can imagine it is the very things that we try to avoid talking about that make up our unfinished emotional business. It is precisely because you may have to face unpleasant memories that it is important you choose a therapist with whom you can feel comfortable and whom you can trust with personal details.

Consider your time in therapy as an opportunity to resolve these emotional issues, and leave it to the therapist to determine whether they are relevant to your current problem. The more emotional baggage you can shed in therapy, the happier and more in control you will feel.

WAYS OF INDUCING HYPNOSIS

It does not really matter whether you are standing up, sitting or lying down when the therapist helps you into hypnosis. However, most hypnotherapists like to make their clients reasonably comfortable, either in a reclining chair or on a couch with the head-end slightly raised.

You have already read about a simple example of hypnosis in the section on self-hypnosis (*see page 30*). Your hypnotherapist may very well use a fairly similar method for the induction. The one thing you are unlikely to see is the swinging watch ...

In the first session the therapist will spend quite a lot of time on the hypnotic induction. This is important because a good-quality hypnosis is the foundation for the sessions to come.

There are hundreds of methods of inducing hypnosis, and it would be beyond the scope of this book to attempt to describe even half of them. However, there are a few aspects that most induction methods have in common, and we shall look at a few of these now.

THE FIXATION METHOD

The therapist will ask you to fix your attention on a particular object in your line of vision and to keep gazing at this object. This can be a spot on the wall, the point of a pencil the therapist holds up in front of you, a rotating spiral, a little light or any other ordinary object that happens to be in front of you. At the same time the therapist may suggest to you that you are getting more relaxed, more comfortable and that, as you relax, your eyelids are getting heavier until you cannot keep your eyes open any more, and that you should allow them to close.

The fixation method is based on getting you to focus on a very narrow point of interest in order to create a kind of mental tunnel vision where outside sounds and everyday thoughts are no longer very important. This concentration helps you to become more aware of yourself, your physical feelings and emotions. As the therapist gives you suggestions for relaxation while you are focusing, a state of comfortable sleepiness is induced that is very peaceful. Depending on your suggestibility, this induction can take anything between two and twenty minutes.

THE CONFUSION METHOD

A typical confusion method may start with the therapist asking you to close your eyes. The therapist might then put a finger on a point between your eyebrows and ask you to 'look' at that point while your eyes remain closed. At the same time you will be asked to count backwards from, say, five hundred to one in your mind, while the therapist suggests that you are getting more and more relaxed with each successive number that you are counting down.

The confusion method uses elements of fixation by directing your attention to a particular part of your body while giving you a mental exercise. Trying to do these two things at the same time overloads the conscious mind so that any suggestions the therapist gives you are much easier to accept. In other words, the conscious mind is being purposely confused or diverted in order to gain better access to the subconscious.

THE RELAXATION METHOD

You have already learned about progressive muscle relaxation (*see page 35*), and this may well form part of the method your therapist uses. Depending on how good a subject you turn out to be, your therapist may give you more or less detailed instructions on focusing on your body and feeling how all the muscles begin to relax. The therapist may also draw your attention to feelings such as warmth or a pleasant tingling, and may include suggestions that with every in-breath you are more relaxed, while with every out-breath you are releasing tension.

In a way, the relaxation method also works with fixation, but the fixation is not maintained for long and instead wanders from one part of the body to the next ('your feet are getting more and more relaxed; feel the warmth and the pleasant tingling in your feet – and now move to your calf muscles ...'). The relaxation effect, again, comes from focusing on yourself, which automatically distracts your attention from external stimuli. This, together with the therapist's suggestions, results in a state of hypnosis that is soothing and relaxing.

At this point let me repeat once again that, no matter which induction method your therapist uses, you will in all likelihood feel quite normal and in no way weird or 'hypnotized'. There is no such thing as a hypnotized feeling. You still know exactly where you are; you can still hear any sounds inside or outside the room. It is just that now all these things become less important because your attention is focused on yourself and your inner physical, mental and emotional experiences. All you will feel is a sense of physical relaxation and a greater feeling of calmness in your mind, so please do not be disappointed if you do not feel like a zombie!

After the induction the therapist will proceed to deepen the initial light hypnosis. A very common method is for the therapist to count backwards, for example from ten to one, while suggesting to you that you feel more relaxed and comfortable with every number that is counted, sinking further and further back into your chair with each successive number.

One way of deepening the hypnosis still further after counting down is by using imagery. The therapist may suggest a pleasant scene such as a sun-drenched beach, an idyllic garden or a comfortable room where you can feel safe and secure. Once the hypnotherapist is satisfied that you are properly in hypnosis, he or she will either start with suggestions concerning your particular problem, or will offer some post-hypnotic suggestions to 'prime' you for entering a deep and comfortable state of hypnosis whenever the therapist says a certain word, such as 'sleep'. In this way the induction time can be considerably reduced next time you have a session.

COUNTING UP

Every hypnotic induction has to be reversed when the session is over. Very often this is achieved simply by the therapist counting upwards again, suggesting that as he or she does so you will become more aware of your surroundings and will come back into the here and now, feeling rested and refreshed.

After you have been counted up and out of hypnosis, the therapist needs to make sure that you are properly out of hypnosis. As hypnosis can be very deeply relaxing, especially for people who are habitually tense and nervous, it can take a while for you to shake that slightly dazed feeling. A simple remedy is to take a few quick breaths and to tense all your muscles sharply a few times to activate the circulation again.

WORKING THROUGH A MEMORY

You will have noticed that throughout this book there have been references not only to finding memories that relate to your immediate problem, but also to working through these memories. What does this mean?

In hypno-analysis you and your therapist would start by finding out which emotional stresses were precursors to your present-day symptoms. If, for example, you suffer from panic attacks and you have done so since the age of 18, it makes sense to go back to the time *before* the first panic attack occurred to look at what was going on in your life at the time. If, however, you are 45 and your panic attacks only started a year ago, there is no immediate need to go all the way back to childhood. Instead, the therapist will first of all concentrate on your memories from 18 months or two years ago to establish whether any particular emotional stresses occurred then. Once the traumatic events, remembered or forgotten, have come to the fore, they can be worked through.

Let us look at a real-life example. Susan's first panic attack occurred at 18, and the emotional stresses before that first panic attack were that Susan had become pregnant at the age of 17, her boyfriend did not want to know and her parents were so ashamed of her that they sent her away to a single mothers' home to have the baby there. They then insisted that Susan give the child up for adoption. As these memories came up during Susan's sessions they brought with them feelings of sadness and upset. Even though Susan remembered these events consciously anyway, she discovered one thing which she had forgotten – that she had had her first panic attack in the home for single mothers, and not, as she had thought previously, once she had left there.

It is at this point that many schools of hypnotherapy stop.

Once the client has recovered the memory together with the emotion that went with the event at the time, the client is considered cured and the present-day symptoms are expected to clear. In some cases it does work like this, but in others, making this emotional connection between now and the past is simply not enough. Insight is useful but not necessarily always the cure.

The therapist has to make sure that memories are not just brought up but that the client is helped to come to terms with them. This entails exploring *all* the feelings that are connected with the original traumatic event. In our example, Susan was helped to explore how she felt about the boyfriend who left at the first sign of her problems, about her parents sending her away because they were concerned more with what the neighbours would say than with their daughter, and also about the loss of her child. In addition to her initial upset, feelings of guilt, anger and resentment now came up. Susan was asked to put these feelings into words and address them in her mind to the person concerned. In hypnosis Susan expressed her disappointment and anger towards her boyfriend and her parents, which she had been too shocked to do at the time. This process helped her get unsettling feelings off her chest, and Susan reported that she felt that the session had had a liberating effect on her and that she felt more in control as a consequence. The panic attacks subsided.

In addition, therapists can help clients further by putting past experiences into a new framework. This can be done by emphasizing the progress a client has made in other areas of life and stressing how the client has dealt successfully with other problems in the past. The therapist might also want to underline how the resolution of each problem can make a person stronger and more effective at dealing with any new stresses in life, and may generally give suggestions for confidence and self-worth. Helping the client work through memories is essential if the therapist is to ensure that the client is not unnecessarily distressed without also being given the inner resources to resolve past problems in a constructive manner, emerging as a stronger person who can go on to lead a symptom-free life.

WHAT HAPPENS IN THE COURSE OF HYPNO-ANALYSIS?

In this section I would like to go into more detail about some of the procedures you can expect when you go for analytical hypnotherapy. An understanding of these processes is useful not just from a general point of view, but also to safeguard against having memories falsely foisted upon you by the therapist.

Some hypnotherapy schools work strictly along Freudian lines. No matter what problem you come with, if analysis is indicated such Freudian practitioners will use free association to access memories that are relevant to your presenting problem. Free association means that once in hypnosis you are encouraged to talk freely about any memories that come to your mind, while the therapist listens and takes notes.

This is an effective method for bringing memories to the surface. Even if you can only think of trivial memories to start with, you soon access more deep-seated material. At the same time, this process of free association can tend to be lengthy because there may be quite a number of memories to be waded through until you get to the recollections that are directly linked to your present problem.

In order to shorten the time it takes to get to important material, the therapist might use a technique commonly known as the 'Tree Shaker'. This involves encouraging you while you are in hypnosis to imagine certain feelings such as being embarrassed, feeling very lonely, feeling guilty or feeling upset, and to link these feelings to something that really happened in your life. As you can see, only unpleasant feelings are addressed by the Tree Shaker technique. This is because emotional problems invariably hark back to negative past experiences. The Tree Shaker allows you to focus on negative feelings straight away, so that the relevant negative memories can emerge sooner rather than later.

It is very important that the Tree Shaker is used in the most general sense by addressing only common emotions. Everybody has at some time in life felt upset, embarrassed or guilty, so mentioning these feelings in the context of the Tree Shaker is fine. Problems start when the therapist includes images such as being surrounded by flames, being immersed in water or being sexually molested. These are not universal experiences; not everyone has gone through these particular traumas in life. If a therapist includes such drastic images in the Tree Shaker, most clients dismiss them as irrelevant to their personal experience. However, some particularly vulnerable or anxious clients may be upset by these images, or may begin to wonder whether something similar has happened to them and they have just forgotten or repressed it. Especially in the case of suggesting sexual interference, this can lead to a false memory. More of this later in the book (*see page 109*).

Another way in which a therapist may start a first hypno-analysis session is by focusing your attention while you are in hypnosis on a particular negative feeling. If, for example, a client suffers from anxiety, the therapist may direct the client to describe the feeling in more detail. This could take the following form:

Therapist: 'And what is it like to have this anxiety?'

Client: 'It's horrible. It's always there. It makes my stomach flutter all the time, I'm always on edge, like waiting for something dreadful to happen.'

Therapist: 'And when you have that horrible feeling that something dreadful is going to happen, are there any other feelings?'

Client: 'I feel so out of control; I cannot cope with anything, I just feel pathetic and useless.'

Therapist: 'And as you are aware of that feeling of being pathetic and useless, let your mind wander back in time and find an earlier memory where you felt like that.'

Client: '. . . it reminds me of how I felt when I was at secondary school when I had that maths teacher. All the kids were scared of her because she would always put you down if you didn't know the answer, and that really made you feel pathetic and useless . . .'

You can see here how the exploration of a feeling is used to link it to a memory which in turn will lead to more memories that the client associates with anxiety. In the example above, the client went on to remember how he had been very scared of this teacher, who frequently picked on him and humiliated him in front of the class. This memory then lead to memories of home life where things were not much better. His mother was very moody and easily upset, so he felt he could not speak to her about his problems. His father only told him to pull himself together, so that he was left alone with his fears of having to face school again the next day. After this particular session, the client reported that he had always remembered his problems at school but had not been aware before that he had not had any support at home.

The reason why hypno-analysis is so useful at discovering forgotten memories is that it works on the emotional, that is the subconscious, level of the mind. As you explore your feelings, those feelings lead to one or two memories, and those memories then start linking up to more recollections. It is like looking at an old photograph. As you see the dress you wore then and your hairstyle, you suddenly find yourself remembering when you wore that dress for the first time or on which occasion the photograph was taken or what happened later that year. One picture leads to another; one memory leads to another memory, and before you know it you have retrieved a wealth of recollections that you have not thought of in years.

It is easiest to understand this process if you imagine that your mind holds all your memories, but that the more recent memories are closer to the surface and therefore more easily accessible. Just like an onion, your memories are arranged in layers, according to their age. When something particularly upsetting occurs in your life, one of two things can happen. Either this upsetting memory is carried along on the top layer over a period of many years, or it is buried deep beneath the lowest layer to hide it away from conscious awareness in order to avoid further upset about it. In the latter case, we speak of *repression*: the memory is still there, but it is tucked away in a far recess of the memory bank.

Once you come across a memory that is related to your present problem, you may experience an emotional reaction and shed some tears, or you may just feel very emotional as you talk about the memory. This is called an *abreaction*; the term means that you have linked an emotion to a time in the past when you first experienced the emotion.

The client in the above example remembered very clearly how he rang home from boarding school to talk to his father about his unhappiness, only to be told by his father that it would all go away, leaving the boy feeling utterly alone and abandoned. The client became very emotional for a minute or two as he re-experienced how awful he had felt at the time.

This abreaction was the turning point in his analysis. He realized that he had been carrying these feelings of anxiety and fear with him ever since then, but that he no longer needed them because they belonged to an earlier time in his life and he could leave them behind.

Another way in which an emotional resolution of past traumatic events can take place is after a session. Emotions may not surface during the session itself but only over the following few days. It is as if the penny only drops after a time delay. Also, an abreaction can be quite a silent affair. Leaving behind a negative emotion by linking it with the original event can happen quietly and is sometimes experienced as a mere sense of relief or a feeling as if a weight has been lifted off your shoulders.

MONITORING YOUR PROGRESS

Once you have started your hypnotherapy sessions, you should see results fairly quickly if you are having suggestion therapy or desensitization therapy. Suggestions should start taking effect within three sessions at the latest; if they do not take hold after two sessions it is usually necessary to look at the underlying causes of the presenting problem. With desensitization, progress will depend also on your commitment to practising relaxation techniques between sessions. Some therapists will give their clients a self-hypnosis tape after the first session (either a recording of the suggestions they have given during the session or a general hypnotic relaxation tape). Provided clients use the tape regularly between sessions, progress can be expected after three to five sessions at the latest, with more substantial results emerging over the next five sessions.

With analytical hypnotherapy it is more difficult to predict when you will first be able to see results. Again, a lot depends on your therapist's skill, but he or she also needs your cooperation to succeed. If you decide to withhold certain memories because you feel embarrassed or awkward talking about them, this will naturally prolong or even make impossible the process of solving your problems. This does not mean that you are expected to do everything by yourself and that you need somehow to manage to produce memories that you have long forgotten. What it does mean is that if you find yourself remembering a past event in one of your sessions, even if it makes you feel a bit uncomfortable you should make every effort to talk about it, if only to say, 'I'm thinking about a memory which I find hard to speak about.' The therapist can then help you to approach the difficult subject safely.

In order to monitor my clients' progress I always make a list of aims with them in their first session of analytical hypnotherapy. I ask them to think for a moment about how they would recognize that they were getting better – if a miracle happened tonight and tomorrow their problems were gone, what would be different? Here are a few examples of lists of aims.

An anxious client's aims could be:

- to wake up in the morning and feel calm
- to stop worrying all the time
- to sleep better
- to be able to concentrate better and remember what I have read
- to stop having palpitations.

An unconfident client's aims could be:

- to be able to say 'no' when I do not have time to do something

- to be able to voice my own opinions

- to stop putting off unpleasant tasks

- finally to return that faulty toaster to the shop

- to apply for a better job.

You can see that all these aims are quite specific, which makes it easy to check them against reality after four to six sessions. This will give you a clear indication of how you are progressing. When an anxious young man finds he has been sleeping better for the last week and that he can remember what he has just read in the papers, his concentration has obviously improved and he has become calmer.

Not all hypnotherapists will make such a list of aims, but that should not stop you from making one for yourself. Formulating the positive outcome that you are striving for keeps you (and the therapist) on track. Jot down at least three items that would tell you that you were improving, and start looking out for positive changes after four or five sessions.

The reason why I first started making a list of aims with my clients was that I noticed how often clients overlooked the fact that they were making progress. Progress can sometimes be so smooth that it is nearly imperceptible. Let me give you an example.

A young man who came to me because he lacked confidence had worked through quite a few memories in his first three sessions of hypno-analysis. When he came for his fourth session and I asked him whether he had noticed any positive changes, he said no. But once I started digging a bit more, it turned out that he had accepted two invitations from colleagues to go out for a drink, something he had never done before. And yet this had not registered as improvement with him because it had seemed so simple. Clients often expect that some amazing inner fireworks will go off when they get better, so that when it all happens quite undramatically they overlook their progress.

Hypnotherapy does not aim to teach you how to 'pull yourself together'; hypnotherapy is about removing inner blocks and obstacles so that you can just go and do the things which you are capable of doing without undue worry or trepidation. As long as only one other person in the world can do what you are trying to achieve in your hypnotherapy sessions, you can do it too. And who knows, you might even find that you are the first person to do something which no one has ever achieved before ...

YOUR QUESTIONS ANSWERED

What if I can't be hypnotized?

You will remember that the only people who cannot be hypnotized are those who are drunk or who are of below-average intelligence. The fact that you have read this book so far already excludes you from the latter category, so don't worry. Just remember that being hypnotized may not feel as you expect it to feel, but that does not mean you are not in hypnosis.

What if I can't remember anything from the past?

Everyone can remember *something* from the past, no matter how unimportant. You may remember what the house looked like where you lived as a ten-year-old; you may remember your school building or parts of your route to school. These are good starting points which will lead on to more memories. If you get stuck, your therapist can help you get back into the memory process.

Are we looking for a deep dark secret in the sessions?

No. A great number of problems go back to events that you remember anyway, but may have forgotten how much they

HOW TO FIND
A REPUTABLE
HYPNOTHERAPIST

Over the last few years there have been some critical reports about hypnotherapy in the media, some concerning certain schools of hypnotherapy, others investigating individual hypnotherapists. Tabloid sensationalism aside, a great number of the concerns voiced were justified and need to be taken seriously.

Hypnotherapy training is still very varied, with courses ranging in length from three months to two years. Some courses are purely on a correspondence basis, without any mandatory practical training. These courses can be good, but only when taken in conjunction with a practical course; after all, you would not want to be operated upon by a surgeon who had only read textbooks and had never worked on real patients. It is relatively easy to help someone else into hypnosis, but it takes a lot of skill to be able to carry on from there. For this, therapists need to practise under supervision to ensure that they become proficient and learn to apply the basic techniques correctly. No correspondence course can provide this type of training.

The length of the course a therapist has done is not necessarily a guarantee that the therapist is good, but it stands to reason that practitioners who have spent six months learning a skill are going to be better qualified than those who have received their qualification after a weekend seminar.

Those hypnotherapists who specialize in analytical hypnotherapy should also have undergone a training analysis during or after their course. A training analysis requires future therapists to go through the same process that they propose to take their clients through later on when they are in practice. During this analysis the trainee therapists need to confront their own problems and emotions and sort them out where necessary. The training analysis should be carried out by an experienced hypnotherapist who has been practising for at least three years. In this way, future clients can be sure that their therapist knows what it feels like to be at the receiving end of hypnotherapy.

Therapist should also be covered by a professional indemnity insurance which covers them in case a lawsuit is brought against them for malpractice. Hypnotherapists who are found to be misusing their position of trust by sexually harassing or molesting clients should certainly be brought to justice and struck off the register of the organization they belong to, but in some cases hysterical clients whose advances have been rejected by the therapist (and yes, it *does* happen) can end up making unfounded allegations of misconduct. Professional indemnity insurance is there for the therapist's own protection, as it is beyond the means of most people to find the money for legal defence in case a matter goes to court. Over the last years, premiums for professional indemnity insurance have come down considerably, which tells us that most practitioners only very rarely need to make use of their insurance.

Professional indemnity insurance is not available to individuals. In order to obtain this insurance a therapist needs to be a member of an approved association.

Over the last ten years there have been a growing number of reports about child sexual abuse. Whereas you would never have heard this topic mentioned at all 20 years ago it has become a widely discussed issue which is even broached by television and film personalities, who speak openly about their own childhood experiences of sexual abuse. This increased media attention may seem to suggest that there is an increase in child sex abuse, but this is not necessarily the correct conclusion to draw. The fact that we hear more about child abuse now than we did ten years ago only indicates that it is no longer a taboo subject and therefore more widely reported, not that it occurs more widely.

We may not know what percentage of adults have been sexually abused as children, but we certainly know that the problem exists and that it can be soul-destroying to any child who has gone through it. Depending on the gravity and frequency of the abuse, the experience can leave lifelong emotional scars and can, in extreme cases, lead to attempts of self-mutilation and suicide. There can be no doubt that having been sexually abused as a child or teenager is one of the most horrendous experiences a person can go through, as anyone will know who has gone through it or who is professionally involved with victims of abuse.

With regard to hypnotherapy, there are two categories of clients who come for treatment: those who have conscious memories of having been sexually abused and want to get help with overcoming the trauma, and those who have no recollection of sexual abuse in childhood. When a client comes with the conscious knowledge of having been abused, the therapist can help him or her work through those past events. However, these particular cases are not under discussion within the False

Memory issue. It is when the client *starts therapy without any memories of having been abused* and comes out of therapy with the conviction that he or she has been abused that the question arises of whether these are genuine memories or whether the therapist has put ideas of sexual abuse into the client's head.

A number of press and television reports have brought the issue of False Memory Syndrome to the attention of the public. In particular the Ramona case in California has received a lot of publicity. Gary Ramona brought an eight million dollar lawsuit against his daughter's therapists for allegedly planting false memories of abuse in her mind. He won the case and was awarded half a million dollars compensation, but his private life was already in ruins. After the allegations he lost his job and his wife left him. In the wake of this and other court cases, professional bodies such as the British Psychological Society and the United Kingdom Council for Psychotherapy have set up working parties to investigate false memories, and various private initiatives have sprung up such as The British False Memory Society and The False Memory Syndrome Foundation of Philadelphia in the United States, to name just two organizations that work with parents who claim to have been wrongly accused.

This is all very confusing for an outside observer. Who is right and who is wrong? How safe is it to undergo hypnotherapy in respect of False Memory Syndrome?

At this point it is important to make a further distinction between two groups of clients. Within that group of people who go into therapy without conscious memories of abuse but who then uncover memories of abuse during therapy, there are those who have been abused but have repressed the memory of that abuse, and there are those who are falsely led to believe by the therapist that they have been abused when no such abuse has happened in reality. Let us deal with the former category first.

The various False Memory groups argue that there is no such thing as repressed memories, the reasoning being that anything as traumatic as sexual abuse cannot possibly be forgotten or repressed. However, it is a well-established fact that repression does happen, and this is not just confined to sexual abuse. A book published recently about American occupation of Britain during the Second World War cites several examples where soldiers, deliberately or involuntarily, suppressed memories. It took one soldier 40 years to remember that he had slit the throat of a German in hand-to-hand combat while on patrol. He had thought it was only a nightmare he had had, until – 40 years later at a divisional reunion – his former platoon commander confirmed that he had done it. Equally there are examples of clients who unexpectedly come across memories of sexual abuse during hypno-analysis and later find a witness who can confirm these memories. Sometimes this is a sibling who witnessed the assault but did not dare speak out at the time; sometimes, the witness is an adult who knew about the abuse but out of weakness or fear did not dare confront the abuser at the time.

In summary, it has to be concluded that as long as there is even only one case in which a memory has been forgotten, then has emerged during therapy and been corroborated by a witness later on, we cannot discount the idea that a human being is capable of suppressing a traumatic memory as a way of coping with an emotional overload.

Sexual abuse happens in secret, and there are rarely any witnesses. We need to be realistic and admit that human wickedness and perversion as well as indifference to other people's suffering do exist, so we need to be very careful about dismissing too easily the notion that repression can occur when a child is subjected to a terrifying experience such as sexual abuse.

False Memory organizations have done some valuable work

112   in examining the theories upon which various schools of psychotherapy and hypnotherapy are based. The main problem that has been identified is that there are schools of psychotherapy and hypnotherapy which believe that the prime cause of all psychological and emotional problems is child sexual abuse, *and that everyone has experienced some form of sexual abuse in childhood* but that most people have repressed these memories. Consequently, according to these schools, the role of the therapist consists in 'helping' the client 'remember' the abuse trauma. It is no wonder that therapists who come from these schools will find what they are looking for simply because they consciously or subconsciously strive to influence the client in that direction. Whatever the client remembers will then be interpreted to fit into the theory. This, of course, is a totally irresponsible way of working with clients and can do immeasurable harm, particularly in conjunction with hypnosis where a person is more suggestible.

It has to be said quite clearly that we can all be brainwashed, with or without hypnosis, given enough time and exposure to certain suggestions, especially if we are in a vulnerable emotional state. Suggestions can be embedded within a question we are asked. A client might recall a time when her father gave her a cuddle when she was 13.

Therapist: 'And how did you feel about it?'
Client: 'I didn't like it.'
Therapist: 'Was he touching you then?'
Client: 'Yes, he was pressing me against him.'

The therapist's question about whether the father was 'touching' the daughter is leading the client into a statement that may create an entirely false picture. It is possible that the father was up to no good, but it is equally possible that the father was just an affectionate man who did not take into account that a growing girl in puberty might feel awkward about physical contact which, as a younger child, she was happy with. It is therefore unacceptable for the therapist to decide for the client, even by inference only, that her father was 'touching' her.

The therapist needs to encourage recall in a neutral manner. If sexual abuse did indeed happen to a client, it will eventually come out without the therapist 'helping' with leading questions or suggestions.

Memories are not always clear, and many clients will recall an event while saying that they are not sure whether it actually happened or whether they dreamed it. Again, it is not the therapist's job to push the client either way. The therapist's task is to help the client come to terms with the memories in an unaided way during sessions.

It is of paramount importance, both in psychotherapy and in hypnotherapy, that no harm is done either to clients or to their relatives. Memories have to be treated with respect, and every effort has to be made to avoid tampering with them, because the agony of the abused child who is faced with denial from the abuser is just as great as the agony of the falsely accused 'abuser'.

CHECKLIST: WHAT TO LOOK OUT FOR

Here is a summary of points you should consider when you decide to go for hypnotherapy treatment.

Before You Make an Appointment
- Ideally, choose a hypnotherapist who has been recommended by someone you know – either a family member, friend or colleague.

- If you cannot get a recommendation, decide first whether you would prefer to see a male or a female therapist.

- Preferably choose a practitioner who has been practising for quite a long time – perhaps you will have seen his or her advertisements over a long period of time?

- Notice how quickly your phone call is answered; this will give you an indication of how professional the therapist is.

- If you are anxious, take a friend for the initial consultation, but do tell the therapist that you want to bring someone along to sit in on your initial meeting.

When You Receive a Brochure
- What are the therapist's qualifications? With what official bodies is he or she a member?

- What are the fees, and are they on a sliding scale for clients who may be less well off?

- For which conditions is the therapist offering treatment? (Not all therapists will treat the whole range of conditions that hypnotherapy can help with.)

- Does the brochure contain a short explanation about the workings of hypnosis?

- Does it contain a brief explanation of whether the therapist does suggestion therapy, desensitization, analytical hypno-therapy and/or any other associated therapies?

When You Go for the Initial Consultation
- Check whether the consultancy room is reasonably quiet. Banging doors and people shouting in the building can disrupt sessions.

- Find out how long the therapist has been in practice.

- If they have been in practice for less than a year, find out whether they are being supervised or if they can at least get advice from a more experienced therapist if they need it.

- Have a look at the diplomas on the wall to inform yourself about the therapist's qualifications. If you have any queries concerning this point, this is the time to ask!

- *Unless you consciously remember having been abused as a child, ask whether the therapist believes that all problems go back to some form of sexual abuse in childhood.* If the answer is 'yes', you are not advised to start with this therapist.

- Find out whether the therapist has professional indemnity insurance.

- Make sure you understand how much you are expected to pay per session and what exactly you are paying for.

- Check how you feel about the therapist. Unless you are quite happy with the information you have and your rapport with the therapist, go away and sleep on it before you commit yourself to anything.

When Your Background History Is Taken
- Expect to be asked personal questions such as whether you have ever had an abortion or miscarriage.

- Be honest about what has happened/is happening in your life.

- Even if your therapist does not take your background history, mention in your first session briefly any past events that might have a bearing on your present problems.

- Before or after your first session, make a list of aims for yourself, unless the therapist has already done so with you. What would tell you that you are getting better? Remember to check your progress against this list after a few sessions.

- Make sure you sit or lie comfortably. It is difficult to relax if your back aches or the chair is digging into your legs.

- Make sure you are warm enough; if not, ask for a blanket.

- Keep an open mind as to how it will feel to be in hypnosis.

- Notice which signs of hypnosis you can detect:

  watery eyes; changes in breathing; feeling very heavy or very light; feeling like you are moulded into the chair; not wanting to move even though you know you could; feeling that time has gone very quickly; feeling that your hands are bloated; experiencing little muscle jerks in your hands, arms, feet or legs.

- If the therapist says or does anything that makes you feel uncomfortable, say something. If it is urgent, say it during the session; if it can wait, say it at the end of the session.

- If there is anything you do not understand, ask at the end of the session.

Vera Peiffer can be contacted at the following address:

P.O. Box 2517
London W5 5LN

USEFUL ADDRESSES

The Atkinson-Ball College of Hypnotherapy and
Hypno-healing
PO Box 70
Southport
Merseyside PR8 3JB
Tel. 01704 576285
Practical and theoretical training in suggestion therapy, pin-point analysis, NLP (Neuro-linguistic Programming) and hypno-healing for students at an advanced level. Teachers work with real-life clients in front of the class to demonstrate the application of what has been taught.

Graduates use the letters MABCH and MCAH (Member of the Corporation of Advanced Hypnotherapy) after their names.

British Hypnosis Research
St Matthews House
1 Brick Row
Darley Abbey
Derby DE22 1DQ
Tel. 01332 541030
Practical and theoretical training in suggestion therapy using

metaphors and NLP (Neuro-linguistic Programming). Lecturers work with real-life clients in front of the class.

Graduates use the letters DipEHP NLP (BHR) after their names.

British Association of Therapeutical Hypnotists
World Federation of Hypnotherapists
3 Clifton Park
Cromer
Norfolk NR27 9BE
Tel. 01263 512046
A correspondence course that is based on taped lectures and practical workshops.

Graduates use the letters MBATh.H. and MWFH after their names.

The British Society of Medical and Dental Hypnosis
42 Links Road
Ashtead
Surrey KT21 2HJ
Tel. 01372 273522
Training with the Society is open only to medical doctors.

Certification of accreditation is given only after two years of practical use of hypnosis.

The Hypnothink Foundation
PO Box 66
Gloucester GL2 9YG
Tel. 01452 731128
A correspondence course which covers suggestion therapy and analytical hypnotherapy, with a practical workshop at the end.

Graduates use the letters DHyp MHF after their names.

London College of Clinical Hypnosis
229a Sussex Gardens
Lancaster Gate
London W2 2RL
Tel. 0171–402 9037

Practical and theoretical training in suggestion therapy, analytical therapy and NLP (Neuro-linguistic Programming).

Graduates refer to themselves as 'Registered Clinical Hypnotherapists'. No designating letters accompany this title.

The London School of Eclectic Hypnotherapy
808A High Road
Finchley
London N12 9QU
Tel. 0181–446 2210

Practical and theoretical training in clinical hypnotherapy (suggestion therapy), analytical hypnotherapy and holistic hypnotherapy to reach Certified Diploma level.

Graduates use the letters MAAT after their names.

The British False Memory Society
Bradford on Avon
Wiltshire BA15 1NA
Tel. 01225 868682

The Society is concerned with researching the False Memory Syndrome, and with helping those who feel that they have been unjustly accused of sexual abuse by someone who has undergone psychotherapy, hypnotherapy or any other treatment where false memories might have been planted by the therapist in the mind of the client.

INDEX

abortion 90
abreaction 29, 101
affirmation 17
agoraphobia 53
analytical hypnotherapy
    (see also hypno-analysis)
    22, 24–30, 102
anger 26, 48–9, 51, 78, 97
animal magnetism 2
anorexia 24, 56, 57
anxiety 19, 24, 27, 43, 50–2,
    54, 58
asthma 14, 24, 78
attention 12
autonomic nervous system
    8–9, 77

background history 90–2
bed–wetting 14
bingeing 24, 56
blood–pressure 10, 77
British Hypnotism Act 39

brochure 87
bulimia 24, 56, 57

cancer 74, 78
case histories
    anxiety 51–2
    asthma 80
    bulimia 59–60
    dental surgery 76
    depression 49–50
    golf 83–4
    obsessive thoughts 72–3
    phantom pain 77
    phobia 5
    premature ejaculation 68–9
    self–worth 64–5
    smoking 45–7
childbirth 14
childhood 9, 26, 39, 48, 63
Chronic Fatigue Syndrome
    (CFS) 78
compulsions 24, 69–73

Of further interest . . .

ENERGIZE YOURSELF

A COMPLETE GUIDE TO RESTORING LOST VITALITY AND STRENGTH

Vera Peiffer

This practical handbook not only looks at the causes of depleted energy, but also suggests ways in which you can recharge your physical and emotional batteries. Vera Peiffer introduces many down-to-earth methods and techniques aimed at achieving this, all of which are highly effective and fun to carry out.

Discover the benefits of vitamins and minerals, detoxifying, rebounding, breathing, stretching, relaxing, meditating, creative visualization, enjoying music, homoeopathy, shiatsu and much, much more.

Ideal for anyone who feels lethargic, listless or who has recently been ill, *Energize Yourself* is essential reading for anyone needing a kick start in life.

PRINCIPLES OF AROMATHERAPY

THE ONLY INTRODUCTION YOU'LL EVER NEED

Cathy Hopkins

Interest in aromatherapy has grown massively over the last few years. Many people are realizing that the therapeutic properties of plants, contained in the oils extracted from them, can improve our health and well-being in many ways. This introductory guide explains:

- what aromatherapy is
- what its origins are
- what essential oils are
- how to use oils for health, beauty and relaxation
- how to find a practitioner

Cathy Hopkins is a long-time practitioner of aromatherapy and a member of the International Federation of Aromatherapists. She is the author of the bestselling *The Joy of Aromatherapy*.

PRINCIPLES OF NLP

THE ONLY INTRODUCTION YOU'LL EVER NEED

Joseph O'Connor and Ian McDermott

Neuro-Linguistic Programming (NLP) is the psychology of excellence. It is based on the practical skills that are used by all good communicators to obtain excellent results. These skills are invaluable for personal and professional development. This introductory guide explains:

- what NLP is
- how to use it in your life personally, spiritually and professionally
- how to understand body language
- how to achieve excellence in everything that you do

Joseph O'Connor is a trainer, consultant and software designer. He is the author of the bestselling *Introducing NLP* and several other titles, including *Successful Selling with NLP* and *Training with NLP*.

Ian McDermott is a certified trainer with the Society of Neuro-Linguistic Programming. He is the Director of Training for International Teaching Seminars, the leading NLP training organization in the UK.

SELF ESTEEM

A COMPLETE COURSE IN:
· DEVELOPING SELF-WORTH · HEALING EMOTIONAL WOUNDS ·
BREAKING SELF-DESTRUCTIVE HABITS
· BUILDING SELF ESTEEM IN OTHERS

Gael Lindenfield

Poor self esteem is at the root of many of our problems. It can sabotage relationships and careers, cause self-destructive behaviour, and can hold us back from achieving our full potential. The beginnings of poor self esteem usually lie far back in our childhoods, but it can be knocked again in our adult life by criticism and trauma.

Gael Lindenfield, bestselling author and leading therapist, has worked with thousands of ordinary people whose lives have dramatically improved after taking her self esteem courses. This book includes practical exercises that you can do in order to help you improve your own self esteem AND that of others.

Use this book to learn how to be:

- Calm, relaxed and confident
- 'At home' with your body
- Self-reliant
- Energetic and purposeful
- Positive and encouraging with children and colleagues

Praise for Gael Lindenfield's work:

'Great for anyone feeling the need for a confidence boost' *TV Times*

'Sensible, practical and exceedingly useful' *Claire Rayner*

THORSONS INTRODUCTORY GUIDE TO HYPNOTHERAPY

Hellmut W.A. Karle

Hypnosis is in increasing use amongst doctors, dentists and psychologists as an additional therapeutic technique, and also there are now many practising hypnotherapists outside of the medical profession.

Hellmut Karle, a clinical and educational psychologist who has used hypnosis for over 30 years, dispels the myths and misconceptions commonly associated with hypnosis and explains the modern techniques of hypnotherapy and how they can be used to help in many different problems – whether of a physical or psychological nature.

Information is given on what to expect of treatment by hypnosis, and there is advice on how to find properly qualified therapists.

ENERGIZE YOURSELF	0 7225 3111 7	£5.99	☐
PRINCIPLES OF AROMATHERAPY	0 7225 3263 6	£4.99	☐
PRINCIPLES OF NLP	0 7225 3195 8	£4.99	☐
SELF ESTEEM	0 7225 3017 X	£5.99	☐
INTRODUCTORY GUIDE TO HYPNOTHERAPY	0 7225 2534 4	£3.99	☐

All these books are available from your local bookseller or can be ordered direct from the publishers.

To order direct just tick the titles you want and fill in the form below:

Name: _____

Address: _____

_____

Postcode: _____

Send to Thorsons Mail Order, Dept 3, HarperCollinsPublishers, Westerhill Road, Bishopbriggs, Glasgow G64 2QT.

Please enclose a cheque or postal order or your authority to debit your Visa/Access account —

Credit card no: _____

Expiry date: _____

Signature: _____

— up to the value of the cover price plus:

UK & BFPO: Add £1.00 for the first book and 25p for each additional book ordered.

Overseas orders including Eire: Please add £2.95 service charge. Books will be sent by surface mail but quotes for airmail dispatches will be given on request.

24–HOUR TELEPHONE ORDERING SERVICE FOR ACCESS/VISA CARD-HOLDERS — TEL: 0141 772 2281.